Emergencies in Pediatric Oncology

Katrin Scheinemann · Allison E. Boyce

Editors

Emergencies in Pediatric Oncology

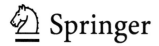 Springer

Editors
Katrin Scheinemann, MD, PhD
Division of Hematology/Oncology
Department of Pediatrics
McMaster Children's Hospital
1200 Main Street West
555 University Avenue
Hamilton, ON L8N 3Z5, Canada
kschein@mcmaster.ca

Allison E. Boyce, RN, BScN
Division of Hematology/Oncology
The Hospital for Sick Children
555 University Avenue
Toronto, ON M5G 1X8, Canada
allison.boyce@sickkids.ca

ISBN 978-1-4614-1173-4   e-ISBN 978-1-4614-1174-1
DOI 10.1007/978-1-4614-1174-1
Springer New York Dordrecht Heidelberg London

Library of Congress Control Number: 2011941609

Printed on acid-free paper

Springer is part of Springer Science+Business Media (www.springer.com)

To our patients and their families who teach us the essence of life every day:
Do not look back in the past or plan for the future; live life to the fullest today!

Preface

The purpose of this book is to give pediatric residents, oncology fellows, and nurses a short and practical guideline to handle the most common emergencies in pediatric oncology. It considers the standard of care for workup of new diagnosis and guidance through emergencies. The multidisciplinary approach of diagnosis and treatment is emphasized through the authors from different disciplines.

We would like to thank our chapter authors for their ideas, time, and knowledge devoted to this project. Special thank you to Donna MacKenzie for the formatting work on the whole book.

We hope that this book will provide answers and guidance for the health care professionals in our field.

Hamilton, ON, Canada   Katrin Scheinemann
Toronto, ON, Canada   Allison E. Boyce

Contents

Contributors

Uma Athale, MD, MSc Division of Hematology/Oncology, McMaster Children's Hospital, Hamilton, ON, Canada

Allison E. Boyce, RN, BScN Division of Hematology/Oncology, Hospital for Sick Children, Toronto, ON, Canada

Anthony K. Chan, MBBS, FRCPC, FRCPath Division of Hematology/Oncology, McMaster Children's Hospital, Hamilton, ON, Canada

Stephanie Cox, RN (EC), MN, NP-Peds Division of Hematology/Oncology, McMaster Children's Hospital, Hamilton, ON, Canada

David C. Hodgson, MD, MPH, FRCPC Department of Radiation Oncology, Princess Margaret Hospital, Toronto, ON, Canada

Paula MacDonald, BScPhm Division of Hematology/Oncology, McMaster Children's Hospital, Hamilton, ON, Canada

Laurence Masson-Côté, MD, FRCPC Department of Radiation Oncology, Princess Margaret Hospital, Toronto, ON, Canada

Barbara-Ann Millar, MBChB (Hons), MRCP, FRCR, FRCPC Department of Radiation Oncology, Princess Margaret Hospital, Toronto, ON, Canada

Normand J. Laperriere, MD, FRCPC, FRANZCR (Hon) Department of Radiation Oncology, Princess Margaret Hospital, Toronto, ON, Canada

Katrin Scheinemann, MD, PhD Division of Hematology/Oncology, McMaster Children's Hospital, Hamilton, ON, Canada

Hanna Tseitlin, BScN, MN, APN Division of Hematology/Oncology, McMaster Children's Hospital, Hamilton, ON, Canada

Chapter 1
Introduction: Pediatric Oncology

Katrin Scheinemann

Keywords APON • Childhood cancer registry • Clinical trials • Hospice • Odilie Schweisguth • Palliative care • Sidney Farber • SIOP • Supportive care

Pediatric oncology can be considered a very young discipline within pediatrics. For a long time, children with cancer were treated by a surgeon, a general practitioner, or a radiologist and the outcome was dismal.

But looking back into history gives an idea about the groundwork.

In the year 1647, Antonj van Leeuwenhoek invented the microscope in Delft (The Netherlands), and suddenly, morphology of human tissue/fluids could be studied [1]. It took over two centuries until Paul Ehrlich from Germany performed and described a blood smear – still a very important diagnostic tool. In 1929, Max Wintote defined the red cell indices (MCV, MCHC, and MCH) which subsequently led to further description of anemia. The first differential blood count was done by Wallace Coulton – the discipline pediatric hematology was born.

However, it needed two pioneers on both sides of the Atlantic Ocean for the development of pediatric oncology: Odilie Schweisguth from France and Sidney Farber from the United States. Odilie Schweisguth was one of the first females to complete a medical degree, which she obtained in 1936 in Paris following a nursing career [2]. She was considered as the first European pediatric oncologist in 1948 and founded the first pediatric oncology ward at the Institute Gustave Roussy (IGR), France's leading cancer center, in 1952. This ward's concept also included a palliative care room as well as a separate room for nurses and physicians. Her research focus was on aftercare and survivorship. She also was a strong advocator for her discipline which led to the initiation of the advanced course on pediatric leukemia and cancer, established in 1954, and the founding of SIOP (International Society of

K. Scheinemann (✉)
Division of Hematology/Oncology, McMaster Children's Hospital,
1200 Main Street West, 555 University Avenue, Hamilton, ON, Canada L8N 3Z5
e-mail: kschein@mcmaster.ca

K. Scheinemann and A.E. Boyce (eds.), *Emergencies in Pediatric Oncology*,
DOI 10.1007/978-1-4614-1174-1_1, © Springer Science+Business Media, LLC 2012

Table 1.1 Major professional organizations in pediatric oncology

Title		Webpage
SIOP	International Society of Pediatric Oncology	www.siop.nl
ASPHO	American Society of Pediatric Hematology/Oncology	www.aspho.org
ASCO	American Society of Clinical Oncology	www.asco.org
GPOH	Society of Pediatric Oncology and Hematology (Germany)	www.krebsinfo.de(webpage available in English)
C^{17}	Council of Children's Cancer and Blood Disorder (Canada)	www.c17.ca
APON	Association of Pediatric Oncology Nurses	www.apon.org
CCRG	Children's Cancer Research Group (UK)	www.ccrg.ox.ac.uk
COG	Children's Oncology Group	www.childrensoncologygroup.org
POGO	Pediatric Oncology Group of Ontario (Canada)	www.pogo.ca

Pediatric Oncology) in 1968. Following the SIOP foundation, multiple other professional organizations have been established, as shown in Table 1.1.

Sidney Farber, on the other hand, worked as a pathologist at the Children's Hospital in Boston [3]. A recent discovery that folic acid stimulated leukemia cell growth and disease progression led to the idea of a clinical trial to use folic acid antagonist for remission achievement. This trial, considered as the first chemotherapeutic trial, got published in the New England Journal of Medicine 1948. Temporary remission was achieved in 10 out of 16 participants. Sidney Farber founded the first comprehensive pediatric oncology treatment center at Boston Children's Hospital. Quite early, he recognized that advancing treatment would only occur with increasing research, so a cancer research foundation was established. He was a strong supporter of multidisciplinary care and invented the multidisciplinary tumor board.

In 1974, the first American pediatric hematology/oncology board exam was held and a new discipline was born [1]. Since then, multiple accredited programs for pediatric hematology/oncology have been established all over the world. International and multi-institutional cooperative therapy groups have been established, and scientific journals in this area have been founded. Multiple professional online information and teaching tools are also available in our days, as outlined in Table 1.2.

Similar to the organizational development on the physician site, an accreditation process on the nursing site took place [4]. Initially, they were referred to as "tumor therapy nurses" and were not allowed to share the diagnosis with their patients or parents. The first oncology nursing and nurse practitioner program were established at St. Jude's Research Hospital in Memphis. The association of pediatric oncology nurses (APON) was founded in 1974. The first certification of pediatric oncology nursing (CPON) took place in 1995.

Each year, over 264,000 children are diagnosed with a malignancy worldwide, with over 80% of them in a low-income country. Presumably, the number is much

Table 1.2 Further online information

Title	Webpage	Content
Cure4Kids	www.cure4kids.org	Continuing medical education focusing on cancer, pediatrics, oncology, and global communication tools
The International Confederation of Childhood Cancer Parent Organizations	www.icccpo.org	Information about parent organization around the world
		Wide range of articles relevant to childhood cancer
Pediatric Oncology Education Material (POEM)	www.pedsoncology education.com	Important aspects of pediatric oncology for health care provider and students
Cure search for Children's cancer	www.curesearch.org	Research, collaboration, clinical trials, and resource material for families

higher as a large number of patients in low-income countries may never get diagnosed and will die without an established diagnosis. Leading diagnoses in high-income countries are leukemias, followed by CNS tumors. Most of the high-income countries have established a childhood cancer registry, keeping track of incidences, potential clusters, treatment, and outcome. Incidences have risen over the past decades, but this is biased by better and more complete registry as well as better diagnostic tools. The biggest hospitals have established subdivisions due to the high number of patients: leukemia/lymphoma, solid tumors, neurooncology, and stem cell transplant. With ongoing treatment advances and the long-term goal of targeted treatment, the prognosis and outcome have changed dramatically. Sixty years ago, only children with a "surgically curable" cancer would have survived their disease. Now, over two-thirds of all children in high-income countries are expected to become long-term survivors – this has lead to a special new subdiscipline of aftercare. Children, adolescents, young adults, and adults are monitored for long-term treatment sequelae, as well as secondary malignancies. But the prognosis has also changed dramatically with the recent advance in supportive care. The availability of blood transfusions and G-SCF, broad-spectrum antibiotics, and the concept of prophylactic antibiotic use have been key players in the reduction of morbidity. The invention of central venous access via port-a-cath or Broviac catheter has made the administration and monitoring of chemotherapy much safer and easier. Finally, different antiemetic drugs have tackled one of the most common but most uncomfortable general side effects: nausea and emesis.

Childhood cancer survivors have now become parents – one of the biggest success stories within medical history. But with the increasing number of childhood cancer survivors, their aftercare also needs to be better organized to monitor their long-term sequelae.

One of the reasons for this success is the effort to treat the majority of children on multicenter clinical trials. All major study groups worldwide (e.g., Children's

Oncology Group) have established and are running clinical trials for all common cancers in childhood. This allows a huge enrollment of patients and plenty of clinical and biological data. The following phases for clinical trial are common:

Phase I: These trials are designed to test the safety, tolerability, pharmacokinetics, and pharmacodynamics of a drug. Phase I studies cannot be offered in all centers as they require special education of the healthcare personnel and intense monitoring.

Phase II: These trials are designed for dosing requirements and drug efficacy based on the results of the phase I study.

Phase III: These studies are multicenter, often randomized, control trials to assess the effectiveness of an investigational arm/drug compared to a known "standard arm." Most clinical trials in pediatric oncology are phase III trials. These trials have a "curative" intent for a specific disease/disease risk group.

But with all this success, we also have to acknowledge that still at least 20% of the children diagnosed with a malignancy are going to die sooner or later in treatment. The early implementation of palliative care can greatly improve symptom management, quality of life, and communication between patients and their family. As palliative care teams are unfortunately undersourced in many hospitals or only get consulted at a later stage, further improvement is necessary over the next years. As more and more patients and their parents have the desire to die at home, the amount of resources in the community has to be increased – a palliative care team covering both in- and outpatient settings would be the ultimate goal. Specialized pediatric hospices are still rare and most adult hospices are only accepting children older than 16 years of age.

References

1. Pearson HA. History of Pediatric Hematology Oncology. Pediatric Research 2002; 52 (6): 979–992
2. Massimo LME. Odilie Schweisguth: Pioneer of European Pediatric Oncology. Pediatric Hematology and Oncology 2003; 20: 75–77
3. Miller DR. A tribute to Sidney Farber – the father of modern chemotherapy. British Journal of Hematology 2006; 134: 20–26
4. Fergusson J. A living legend in pediatric oncology nursing – Jean Fergusson. Journal of Pediatric Oncology nursing 2001; 18 (5): 229–238

Chapter 2
Initial Management of New Diagnosis

Katrin Scheinemann

Keywords Compression syndrome • Electrolyte supplements • Febrile neutropenia • Flow cytometry • Hemorrhage • Hyperleukocytosis • IV hydration • Leukapheresis • Leukostasis • Lymphadenopathy • Pancytopenia • Rasburicase • Renal failure

Initial Contact

While solid tumors and brain tumors often get referred to pediatric surgery and neurosurgery, children with pancytopenia, blasts on peripheral smear, or lymphadenopathy are often referred directly to pediatric oncology.

As these referrals are made by family physicians or pediatricians who potentially have never seen such a case before, guidance is needed for the initial contact.

The following points should be considered:

1. Patient's name and contact information.
2. Age of the patient.
3. History of current illness.
4. Recent blood work:

   Date?
   Exact values?
   Peripheral blood smear?
   Chemistry available?

K. Scheinemann (✉)
Division of Hematology/Oncology, McMaster Children's Hospital,
1200 Main Street West, 555 University Avenue, Hamilton, ON, Canada L8N 3Z5
e-mail: kschein@mcmaster.ca

K. Scheinemann and A.E. Boyce (eds.), *Emergencies in Pediatric Oncology*,
DOI 10.1007/978-1-4614-1174-1_2, © Springer Science+Business Media, LLC 2012

5. When was the patient last seen (delay between taking blood sample and reporting from the outside laboratory)?
6. Last clinical exam?
7. Any other additional test performed? X-ray, etc.?

Upon obtaining this information, a decision has to be made as to how quickly (immediately vs. the next day(s)) and where (ER vs. outpatient clinic vs. direct admission to the inpatient ward) the patient needs to be seen. It is the responsibility of the referring physician to inform the parents about the potential diagnosis of a malignancy and provide information about the next step including the contact person of the referring hospital.

Arrival and First Steps in the Hospital

Upon arrival in the hospital, it is important that the patient/family will be seen as soon as possible by a pediatric oncologist. First, it will help to start a good and trustful relationship as families will have many questions which can only be answered by pediatric oncology. Second, it will help to get the necessary investigations ordered in a timely manner without delays or misses. Third, a quick clinical assessment will help facilitate the further care of the patient and decrease early morbidity.

The following blood work should be ordered:

1. CBC, including differential
2. Peripheral blood smear – to be reviewed by the lab technician and the hematopathologist and/or pediatric oncologist
3. Reticulocyte count
4. Dependent on the white cell count, flow cytometry from peripheral blood should be ordered (not possible with low counts)
5. Electrolytes (Na, K, Cl, PO_4, Mg, Ca)
6. Kidney function test (BUN, creatinine)
7. Bilirubin and liver function test (AST, ALT)
8. Tumor lysis blood work (uric acid, LDH) [please see Chap. 3 for further information]
9. Coagulation screen (PTT, INR) – important for further procedures
10. CMV serology – important to know patient's status prior to the first blood product transfusions

The patient should be started on IV hydration – important to use only normal saline as IV solution. The amount of fluid will be determined by the patient's clinical status and the blood work results. If the patient is febrile, blood cultures should be taken, and the patient should be started on broad spectrum antibiotics as per the institutional febrile neutropenia protocol. Other culture samples such as urine culture or NPS should only be considered with clinical symptoms.

The clinical exam should include at least the following points:

1. Heart – listen for murmurs due to anemia, cardiac effusion
2. Respiratory system/chest – infection, respiratory distress with positioning, pleural effusion
3. Skin – for signs of bleeding including mouth, nose, and ears
4. Abdomen – hepatosplenomegaly, other palpable masses
5. General lymphadenopathy
6. Male patients' testes – for possible malignant infiltration
7. Hydration status
8. Any signs of sepsis without fever – peripheral perfusion and pulses, extremity temperature
9. Other sites of infection – cut, bitten, ingrown toenail, teeth
10. Other "lumps and bumps" – e.g., chloroma in AML
11. Neurological status including fundoscopy
12. Joints and bones – if there was history of joint or bone pain.

Please keep in mind that most of these patients are quite sick and are not feeling well – so please be as gentle and thorough at the same time. Explain to the patient and parents what you are looking for throughout the exam.

Additional testing besides clinical exam and blood work is needed:

1. Chest X-ray, two views – Is there mediastinal mass or infection?
   Please do not lay the patient flat if there are any concerns about respiratory distress prior to the chest X-ray [please see Chap. 4 for further information]
2. U/S testes if concern about malignant infiltration
3. U/S abdomen – hardly necessary, clinical hepatosplenomegaly does not need to be confirmed
4. CNS imaging – only necessary with clinical symptoms/concerns
5. Bone/joint X-ray – dependent on clinical symptoms

With all of these results, the immediate management and risk of the patient will be determined.

The following points should be considered until final diagnosis (bone marrow aspiration/biopsy) is made:

1. IV fluids with normal saline – at least at one-and-a-half at least fluid maintenance, but needs to be increased depending on total white cell count and hydration status
2. No electrolyte supplements should be added unless patient has clinical symptoms
3. Adequate balance monitoring including weight
4. Repeat blood work – frequency will be determined by previous results
5. Blood product transfusion – please consider the need for blood product transfusion carefully as PRBC will increase viscosity and with this morbidity. Blood products should only be transfused either for procedures or for clinical symptoms, e. g., bleeding or signs of acute cardiac failure
6. NPO orders for procedure
7. Consents for procedure and tissue samples
8. Treatment of hyperuricemia [please see Chap. 3 for further information]

Management of Hyperleukocytosis

A high initial white cell count will require immediate intervention and careful monitoring. A white cell count over 100×10^9 per L is defined as hyperleukocytosis. Hyperleukocytosis is more often observed in AML (up to 25%) compared to ALL (10%) and can be seen quite often in infants [1]. The early morbidity (20–40%) and mortality risk with an increased white cell count is higher in AML compared to ALL as the blasts are bigger in size and "stickier" to each other and the endothelium [2]. This phenomenon together with leukostasis is considered as the underlying pathomechanism.

Clinically, the following presentations are possible:

1. Neurologic (stroke, headache, blindness, altered level of consciousness)
2. Respiratory (hypoxia, dyspnea)
3. Hemorrhagic (CNS, GI, pulmonary)
4. Renal failure
5. Metabolic (tumor lysis syndrome)

Patients with symptomatic hyperleukocytosis have a higher risk of morbidity and mortality.

Treatment principles can be summarized as the following:

1. Close observation and monitoring (consider ICU admission)
2. Fluids should be increased to 1.5–2× maintenance with close monitoring of output
3. Correct coagulopathy (plt > $30–50 \times 10^9$ per L, FFP and cryoprecipitate as needed)
4. Avoid PRBC transfusion – if necessary due to clinical symptoms, use a dose of 5 mL/kg
5. Tumor lysis precaution/treatment
6. Reduce white cell count:

   • Early start of chemotherapy
   • Leukapheresis

Leukapheresis

As leukapheresis is a resource-intense procedure with a lot of risks, the decision to proceed has to be made early including all considerations. As all evidence is based on retrospective studies, no clear guidelines are established. Also, with the implementation of rasburicase, the value of leukapheresis is under discussion. Certainly, in patients with symptomatic hyperleukocytosis, it should be considered. The goal is to reduce the total white cell count by 50% or < 100×10^9 per L [3].

As the implementation requires some planning, the decision has to be made as early as possible:

1. PICU admission for close monitoring and central line
2. Pheresis nurse on call
3. Blood bank – volume needed should be calculated prior to contact, platelet transfusion

The needed blood volume needs to be calculated and ordered by the pediatric oncologist – pheresis nurse can help if no institutional guidelines are available
Blood volume calculation:

1. Reconstituted whole blood (with FFP) matches to hematocrit of the patient
2. Close monitoring of platelet count will require repeat transfusions
3. "Double blood volume processing:"

- Infants: 100 mL/kg
- 1–10 years: 80 mL/kg
- >10 years: 70 mL/kg

As leukapheresis is a risky procedure, careful monitoring of the side effects is necessary. Despite the fact that the patient is in the PICU, regular visits from the pediatric oncologists through the procedure are required:

1. Electrolyte imbalance
2. Hemorrhage
3. Respiratory failure
4. Renal failure
5. Allergic reaction to blood product
6. Bleeding from central line site

Depending on the reduction of the white cell count, more than one round of leukapheresis is needed. Diagnosis should not be delayed through the procedure as with the high-white-cell/blast-count flow cytometry and molecular cytogenetics can be performed from peripheral blood. Diagnostic lumbar puncture should wait until the completion of leukapheresis, adequate platelet count, and no coagulopathy.

Solid Tumors/Brain Tumors

As previously mentioned, patients with a suspicion of a solid or brain tumor are often referred to the pediatric surgeon and neurosurgeon. As diagnosis in almost all cases is pathology dependent, the first step is to get a tissue sample plus/minus tumor removal as soon as possible.

Pediatric oncology is getting involved earlier or later depending on the underlying tumor type. Early involvement will have the advantage of closing the gap

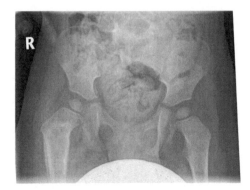

Fig. 2.1 Initial X-ray: Lytic lesion in the right femur

between the biopsy and when the pathology results are available. Further staging investigations or basic organ function tests could be performed throughout the waiting time. Also, patients and their parents will greatly benefit from early involvement of a pediatric oncology social worker to decrease the stress and to implement any paperwork that may be needed (i.e., for financial assistance).

The risk of tumor lysis syndrome is much lower, but still an assessment is necessary. On the other hand, the risk of compression syndrome is higher and will require adequate monitoring. Depending on the patient's clinical status and the underlying malignancy, a discharge between the initial surgical procedure and the disclosure meeting is possible.

Case 1
A 23-month-old boy was brought in with a 4–5-week history of difficulty in weight bearing, wherein the boy only crawled and refused to walk. Admitted to the hospital with right hip pain and fever, X-ray showed a lytic lesion, and he was started on antibiotics. Upon referral to orthopedic surgery, a biopsy of the lytic lesion was performed which revealed a negative gram stain but lots of small round blue cells. Subsequently, a bone marrow aspiration was done which established the diagnosis of pre-B-ALL (Figs. 2.1 and 2.2).

Case 2
A 34-month-old boy presented with lymphadenopathy, on left site of his neck. A course of antibiotics did not decrease the size; instead it was increasing. A referral to an ENT surgeon was made, who performed a biopsy. As the pathology revealed small round blue cell tumor, patient was referred to pediatric oncology. Following re-biopsy and staging investigations, patient was diagnosed with stage IV neuroblastoma (Fig. 2.3).

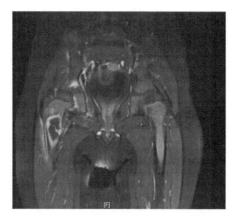

Fig. 2.2 MRI pelvis: Enhancing mass lesion in the proximal diaphysis of the right femor, associated with periostitis surrounding soft tissue edema and enhancement of the adjacent femoral muscles

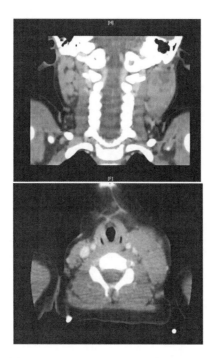

Fig. 2.3 CT neck: Large inhomogeneous mass left side of the neck with lymphadenopathy displacing the left jugular vein. Irregular calcifications within the mass

References

1. Eguiguren JM, Schell MJ, Christ WM, Kunkel K, Rivera GK. Complications and outcome in childhood acute lymphoblastic leukemia with hyperleukocytosis. Blood 1992; 79: 871–875
2. Porcu P, Farag S, Marcucci G, Cataland SR, Kennedy MS, Bissell M. Leukocytoreduction for acute leukemia. Therapeutic apheresis 2002; 6 (1): 15–23
3. Haase R., Merkel N., Diwan O., Elsner K., Kramm CM. Leukapheresis and exchange transfusion in children with acute leukemia and hyperleukocytosis. A single center experience. Klinische Paediatrie 2009; 221: 374–378

Chapter 3
Tumor Lysis Syndrome

Hanna Tseitlin

Keywords Allopurinol • Aluminum hydroxide • Calcium gluconate • Cardiac arrhythmias • Creatinine clearance • Cytotoxic therapy • Diuresis • Hyperhydration • Hyperkalemia • Hyperphosphatemia • Hyperuricemia • Hypocalcemia • Rasburicase • Renal insufficiency • Tumor lysis syndrome

Definition of Tumor Lysis Syndrome

Tumor lysis syndrome (TLS) is a life-threatening condition that results from the rapid destruction of malignant cells in bulky, rapidly proliferating tumors or in highly chemo- and radiotherapy-sensitive disease. Consequently, the cellular content is released into the bloodstream, and the condition becomes associated with electrolyte imbalances such as hyperkalemia, hyperphosphatemia, hyperuricemia, and hypocalcemia (Table 3.1).

Cellular damage leads to the release of nucleic acid, which is in turn catabolized to hypoxanthine, xanthine, and finally uric acid, thus resulting in hyperuricemia. Hyperphosphatemia, on the other hand, results from rapid cellular release of phosphate, where in malignant cells, intracellular phosphate levels can be up to four times higher than in normal cells. As a result of the inability of the tubular transport mechanisms to clear out excess phosphate, an increase in serum phosphate levels can lead to the precipitation of calcium–phosphate binding in the renal tubules. This causes an exacerbation of renal sequelae and can result in renal

H. Tseitlin (✉)
Division of Hematology/Oncology, McMaster Children's Hospital,
1280 Main Street West, Hamilton, ON, Canada L8S 4K1
e-mail: tseitlin@hhsc.ca

K. Scheinemann and A.E. Boyce (eds.), *Emergencies in Pediatric Oncology*,
DOI 10.1007/978-1-4614-1174-1_3, © Springer Science+Business Media, LLC 2012

Table 3.1 Definitions of laboratory abnormalities [1–5]

Element	Absolute value	Change from baseline
Uric acid (Urate)	≥450 μmol/L or 8 mg/dL	25% Increase
Potassium (K)	≥6 mmol/L or 6 mg/L	25% Increase
Phosphate (P)	≥2.1 mmol/L (or ≥ age-appropriate ULN)	25% Increase
Calcium (Ca)	≤1.75 mmol/L	25% Decrease
Azotemia	≥1.5 times upper limit of normal	25% Increase

failure. Calcium–phosphate binding can further contribute to decreased serum calcium levels, which may lead to hypocalcemia with possible clinical features of muscle cramping and cardiac arrhythmias. Another essential intracellular component that gets released into the blood stream during cell disintegration is potassium. Increased serum potassium levels may result in hyperkalemia, which is often exacerbated by the already compromised renal system and can lead to cardiac irregularities such as arrhythmias, fibrillation, ventricular tachycardia, and cardiac arrest. It can also trigger neuromuscular effects such as muscle cramping and paresthesia [1, 2].

Due to the fast progression and serious clinical implications, it is associated with high morbidity and mortality [2].

Incidence

The incidence of TLS reported in the literature varies between 3 and 25%, depending on the diagnosis [1–4]. Laboratory TLS is present in about 20% of patients, where the clinical presentation of TLS happens in about 3–5% of patients [1–4]. In most cases, the syndrome is associated with the diagnosis of hematological malignancy such as acute lymphoblastic leukemia, Burkitt's lymphoma, and acute myeloid leukemia. Although rare, there are reported cases of TLS in patients with solid tumors. In most cases, it is associated with large, highly proliferative tumors that are chemosensitive. TLS in patients with solid tumors tends to be unpredictable in its characteristics and timing. As a result, the mortality rate associated with TLS in patients with solid tumors is as high as 36% [1–3] (Tables 3.2 and 3.3).

Table 3.2 High risk factors (1) Type of malignancy, tumor burden, (2) WBC count, (3) Uric acid level at the base line, (4) Renal function at the time of diagnosis

Type of malignancy	Tumor burden	WBC count	Uric acid level at baseline	Renal function at time of diagnosis
Burkitt's lymphoma	Bulky disease	Elevated WBC	≥450 μmol/L	Serum creatinine
Acute lymphoblastic	(>10 cm)	(>25,000	or 8 mg/dL	≥1.5 times
leukemia	Elevated LDH	per μL)		upper limit of
Lymphoblastic	(>2 times ULN)			normal
lymphoma				
Large cell lymphoma				

Table 3.3 Risk group categories for development of TLS [1, 2]

Low risk group	Intermediate risk group	High risk group
Solid tumors except for Neuroblastoma and Germ Cell tumors	Neuroblastoma Germ Cell tumors	Burkitt's lymphoma/leukemia
AML with WBC ≤ 25,000 And LDH < 2 × ULN	AML with WBC ≤ 25,000 and LDH ≥ 2 × ULN	ALL with WBC < 100,000 and LDH ≥ 2 × ULN
	AML with WBC ≥ 25,000 < 100,000 and LDH ≥ 2 × ULN	ALL with WBC > 100,000
	ALL with WBC < 100,000 and LDH < 2 × ULN	

Presentation

Two types of TLS have been classified by Cairo and Bishop [3]: laboratory (LTLS) and clinical (CTLS).

Features of the laboratory type (LTLS):

- Two or more laboratory findings:

  - That are more than or less than the normal levels at the time of presentation
  - Or change of 25% from the baseline within 3 days before or 7 days after start of therapy

  Features of the clinical type (CTLS):

- All the LTLS conditions plus two or more clinical features:

  - Renal insufficiency
  - Cardiac arrhythmias
  - Seizures (Fig. 3.1)

Preexisting renal impairment should be taken into account when establishing risk category for each individual patient. In the presence of renal compromise at the time of diagnosis, the risk group should be upstaged to the next higher level, i.e., low-risk patient with uremia or hyperuricemia at the time of diagnosis would be classified as an intermediate risk.

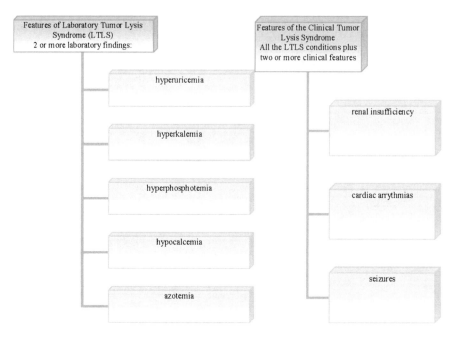

Fig. 3.1 Signs and symptoms of LTLS vs. CTLS. [1, 3, 4]

Clinical Manifestations

Clinical symptoms may present at the time of diagnosis but more commonly appear 12–72 h after initiation of cytotoxic therapy [1]. Clinical symptoms of TLS vary andmay include, but are not limited to [1–5]:

Gastrointestinal symptoms:

- Nausea
- Vomiting

Renal symptoms:

- Reduced urinary output
- Edema
- Fluid overload

Cardiac abnormalities:

- Cardiac dysrhythmias
- Congestive heart failure

Neuromuscular symptoms:

- Lethargy
- Muscle cramping

- Tetany

  Sudden death

TLS Treatment and Supportive Care

Supportive care is a key in prevention and treatment of TLS. It consists of hyperhydration, electrolyte monitoring, and diuresis in the absence of obstructive uropathy. At the time of presentation, supportive measures listed below should be undertaken [1–5]:

- Establish IV access to maintain adequate hydration.
- Obtain baseline blood work as listed below. This is suggested but not limited to the list:
  - CBC with differential
  - Electrolytes should include sodium (Na), potassium (K), phosphate (P), calcium (Ca), and magnesium (Mg)
  - Renal function: urea (BUN) and creatinine
  - Uric acid
  - Liver function should include transaminases (AST and ALT), bilirubin (total and direct), LDH, and albumin

The frequency of blood work should be determined once baseline results are available and patient's risk factors are established. All patients, regardless of their risk factors and the initial results, should have blood work drawn at least once every 24 h. The frequency of blood work should be increased up to every 4–6 h, if there are abnormalities at baseline or if high risk factors have been identified. Repeated blood work should include:

1. CBC with differential
2. Electrolytes: sodium, potassium, phosphate, calcium, and magnesium
3. Renal functions: BUN and creatinine
4. Serum uric acid, LDH, and albumin

Other studies could be added to the list as clinically indicated. Daily monitoring should include:

- Weight
- Fluid balance
- Cardiac monitoring
  - The rate of hydration to be calculated is based on 2–3 $L/m^2/day$ with the goal to maintain urinary output between 80 and 100 $mL/m^2/h$ or between 60 and 80% of the input.
  - In the absence of signs of obstructive uropathy or hypovolemia, diuretics could be used to maintain adequate urinary output. Loop diuretics are the drug of choice in those cases when diuresis is required.

– Although creatinine is often used for monitoring renal function and identifying possible damage, it is a poor indicator of the acute kidney damage. Creatinine clearance or GFR would be more reliable; however, it would require a 24-h urine collection. For a quick estimation of renal function, a calculated GFR should be used based on the Schwartz formula [5]:

$$0.55 \times length(cm) \times 88.4 \,/ \, serum \; creatinine \; (mg/dl)$$

– Dialysis should be considered in patients with persistent hyperkalemia and hyperphosphatemia, symptomatic hypocalcemia, severe acidosis, fluid overload not responsive to diuretics, and in cases of symptomatic uremia such as pericarditis and encephalopathy [5].

There are two pharmacological agents that are available for prevention and treatment of hyperuricemia: allopurinol and rasburicase. Allopurinol is a xanthine oxidase inhibitor that arrests conversion of hypoxanthine and xanthine into uric acid. Although allopurinol reduces uric acid production, it may potentially lead to accumulation of xanthine that is even less soluble than uric acid in the urine. Subsequently, xanthine may precipitate in the kidneys, instigating nephropathy; therefore, renal functions should be closely monitored. Allopurinol should be administered at a dose of 10 mg/kg/day, divided every 8– 24 h. The maximum dose should not exceed 800 mg/day [6, 7].

Rasburicase is an enzyme – urate oxidase – that is found in many mammalian species but not in humans. Its main function is to catabolize existing uric acid to allantoin, which is four to five times more soluble than uric acid. Studies done by Navolanic and colleagues [8] demonstrated that administration of single-dose rasburicase leads to dramatic reduction of uric acid within 4 h after administration even in patients with baseline hyperuricemia. Although rasburicase is highly effective in treating hyperuricemia, its use should be carefully considered due to high cost therefore should be reserved for high risk patients, patients with uric acid elevation at baseline and signs of renal impairment. Rasburicase should be administered at a dose of 0.05–0.2 mg/kg/dose as a single dose and repeated when clinically indicated. G6PD assay blood work should be obtained in all patients where the status is not known since rasburicase is contraindicated in patients with G6PD deficiency. In the process of uric acid destruction, there is a release of H_2O_2, an oxidant that can lead to hemolysis in patients with G6PD [6–11].

Given that the goal of TLS treatment is prevention, patients identified as low risk should be started on allopurinol with the intention of preventing accumulation of uric acid. Intermediate-risk group patients should also be started on allopurinol; however, a close monitoring schedule should be followed, and in the event of hyperuricemia, despite the administration of allopurinol, rasburicase may be considered.

Patients in the high-risk group or those upgraded to this risk group due to hyperuricemia could be treated with rasburicase as a first-line therapy (Fig. 3.2).

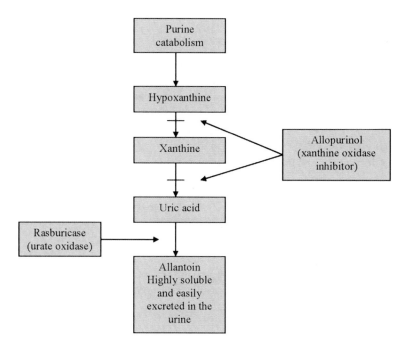

Fig. 3.2 Pharmacological treatment of hyperuricemia: [2, 4]

Treatment of Hyperkalemia

As mentioned earlier, the key in treating TLS is prevention; thus, all intravenous or oral administration of potassium should be discontinued.

Cardiac monitoring should be implemented for early identification of cardiac manifestations such as EKG changes and dysrhythmias. In asymptomatic patients with mild elevation in potassium <6 mmol/L, conservative intervention like hyperhydration and cardiac monitoring would be sufficient as a first-line therapy. In patients with moderate elevation of 6–7 mmol/L that remain asymptomatic, sodium polystyrene sulfonate at 1 gm/kg/dose with 50% sorbitol every 6 h orally.

In patients with severe elevation of potassium > 7 mmol/L and in symptomatic patients, more aggressive treatment modalities should be implemented to counteract hyperkalemia and its effects. Calcium gluconate could be administered to antagonize the cardiac membrane effect of hyperkalemia at a dose of 50–100 mg/kg iv as a single dose. Insulin temporarily influxes potassium back into the cells, thus lowering serum concentration; it could be administered at 0.1 IU/kg with 25% dextrose solution at 2 mL/kg iv. Another temporary but very effective and readily available treatment for hyperkalemia is β-2 antagonists such as nebulized albuterol 10–20 mg that translocates potassium into the cells [2, 5, 6].

Treatment of Hyperphosphatemia

As with hyperkalemia, hyperhydration should continue to promote renal excretion of excess phosphate. All oral and intravenous phosphate supplementation should be discontinued and treatment implemented at serum levels of phosphate ≥ 2.1 mmol/L or at the levels that are $\geq$ age-appropriate upper limit of normal. Phosphate-binder aluminum hydroxide is the most commonly used agent for treatment of hyperphosphatemia. Aluminum hydroxide is administered at a dose of 50–100 mg/kg/day in divided doses every 6 h orally or via nasogastric tube [2, 5, 6].

Sevelamer hydrochloride is another phosphate binder that is available for use in children with hyperphosphatemia. It comes in a pill form and thus has an advantage over aluminum hydroxide, which is only available in the liquid form and poorly tolerated by many children due to its texture and flavor. Sevelamer could be administered at a dose of 400 mg twice daily and could be used anywhere from 1–7 days depending on patient response [12].

In children that present with severe hyperphosphatemia, hemodialysis remains the treatment of choice and requires consultation of a nephrologist [2, 6].

Treatment of Hypocalcemia

Hypocalcemia in TLS is usually a consequence of elevated serum phosphate levels; therefore, treatment of hyperphosphatemia would subsequently reduce calcium–phosphate binding and correct hypocalcemia. The treatment of hypocalcemia should be reserved for patients that exhibit clinical symptoms such as muscle cramping, tetany, seizures, prolonged QT, and cardiac dysrhythmias. Hypocalcemia could be treated with administration of calcium gluconate at 50–100 mg/kg iv with careful cardiac monitoring. Use of calcium gluconate should be carefully considered in the presence of elevated serum phosphate levels because of the risk of increased precipitation and potential obstructive uropathy [2, 6].

Summary

Tumor lysis is a potentially life-threatening condition that is timed with the diagnosis of malignancy and initiation of cytotoxic treatment. Clinical signs and symptoms can vary from patient to patient; hence, close monitoring should be implemented at the time of diagnosis. Risk factors for each patient should be thoroughly reviewed and risk category established prior to treatment initiation. Given that prevention of TLS is the best treatment modality, hyperhydration and surveillance are vital to managing electrolyte abnormalities. Supportive care such as cardiac monitoring, frequency of blood work, and symptoms management should be based on risk category. Additional pharmacological treatments should be instigated at the first laboratory signs of TLS in the attempt to prevent the development of clinical TLS.

Case Study 1

A 13 year-old-boy presented to the Emergency Department with 5 days history of diarrhea, weight loss, nausea, and increased abdominal distension. On examination, there was abdominal distension and tenderness over right upper quadrant, epigastric, and left upper quadrant areas consistent with ascites. CT showed evidence of extensive lymphadenopathy with ascites and bilateral pleural effusion. The boy was admitted for further investigation with clinical picture suggestive of possible lymphoma. A bone marrow aspiration and biopsy were performed that confirmed the diagnosis of Burkitt's lymphoma.

Initial blood work consisted of CBC with differential and chemistry. CBC was within normal limits. Initial chemistry was also normal, with K at 4.1 mmol/L, P at 0.79 mmol/L, urea at 7.9 mmol/L, with normal creatinine at 72 μmol/L, and normal Ca at 2.24 mmol/L. LDH was abnormally elevated at 1,876 U/L. At the time of presentation, uric acid was already elevated at 1,227 μmol/L.

Examining risk factors for this patient, it is obvious that he would be considered as a high risk for TLS due to the diagnosis of Burkitt's lymphoma and in the presence of elevated LDH.

Since the diagnosis was not immediately available, and considering an elevated uric acid level at the time of diagnosis, the patient was started on allopurinol. Blood work was ordered to be repeated every 6 h, and he was admitted to ICU in the anticipation of TLS.

The Children's Oncology Group treatment protocol for Burkitt's lymphoma includes rasburicase that has been integrated due to high probability of tumor lysis in children diagnosed with this disease. As such, the patient has received initial dose of rasburicase and was started on methylprednisolone as per induction course of the protocol.

Please see his blood work at starting therapy (Table 3.4).

Consequently, the patient started having wide complex tachycardia despite Kayexalate, sodium bicarbonate, calcium chloride, dextrose, and insulin administration. Cardiac output was lost for about 20–30 s, and the patient was showing pattern of ventricular tachycardia requiring defibrillation. Furthermore, his urinary output has decreased to 0.5 mL/kg/h, and his urea and creatinine were elevated over two times ULN. In view of risk of uric acid and calcium phosphate crystallization causing tubular obstruction and increasing urea and creatinine values, dialysis was initiated. Three days after the initiation of dialysis, electrolyte imbalances were controlled, and urea and creatinine returned to normal. Subsequently, the patient was transferred to the inpatient unit for continuous recovery and completion of induction chemotherapy.

Table 3.4 Blood work result

Laboratory value	Baseline	4 h into chemotherapy treatment	5 h into chemotherapy treatment	6 h into chemotherapy treatment
Potassium	4.1	8.7	8.8	7.5
Phosphate	1.92	4.09	4.42	3.49
Calcium	2.29	2.66	1.2 (ionized)	
Creatinine	88	131	168	122
Urea	5.02	11.6	22.5	14.2

Table 3.5 Blood work result

Values	Days of therapy			
	1	2	3	4
Potassium	4.0 mmol/L	4.2 mmol/L	4.3 mmol/L	4.1 mmol/L
Phosphate	1.46 mmol/L	1.29 mmol/L	1.26 mmol/L	1.27 mmol/L
Calcium	2.12 mmol/L	2.15 mmol/L	2.18 mmol/L	2.15 mmol/L
Creatinine	83 μmol/L	68 μmol/L	57 μmol/L	61 μmol/L
Urate	220 μmol/L	304 μmol/L	113 μmol/L	84 μmol/L
LDH	325 U/L	278 U/L	267 U/L	208 U/L

Case Study 2

A 17-year-old male presented to his family physician with complaints of ankle pain, back pain, and night sweats. A complete blood count was obtained and some abnormal cells suspicious for leukemia were identified; consequently, he was admitted to the hospital to complete diagnostic workup. The diagnosis was confirmed, and he commenced therapy 5 days after initial presentation.

At the time of presentation, his blood work consisted of WBC 20 g/L, Hb 82 g/L, and platelets 82,000 g/L. His chemistry consisted of potassium 4.1 mmol/L, phosphate 1.5 mmol/L, calcium 2.44 mmol/L, creatinine 84 μmol/L, urate 434 μmol/L, and LDH 322 U/L. Based on those results and the diagnosis of acute lymphoblastic leukemia, he was classified as low risk for TLS.

As mentioned earlier, prevention is the key in managing tumor lysis; therefore, he was started on hyperhydration and allopurinol. The results of his chemistry panel for 4 days after initiation of chemotherapy are shown in Table 3.5.

As evident from the table, all indices associated with TLS remained stable and within normal limits for age 4 days into initiation of therapy; allopurinol and hyperhydration were discontinued on day 7 of therapy, and he was discharged home on day 10 of induction.

References

1. Cairo, M.S., Coiffler, B., Reiter, A. and Younes, A. Recommendations for the evaluation of risk and prophylaxis of tumor lysis syndrome (TLS) in adults and children with malignant disease: an expert TLS panel consensus. British Journal of Hematology, 2010;149; 578–586
2. Coiffler, B., Altman, A., Pui, C-H. and Cairo, M.S. Guidelines for the management of pediatric and adult tumor lysis syndrome: an evidence-based review. Journal of Clinical Oncology. 2008; 26(16), 2767–2778
3. Cairo, M.S. and Bishop, M. Tumor lysis syndrome: new therapeutic strategies and classification. British Journal of Haematology. 2004; 127; 3–11
4. Mughal, T.I., Ejaz, A.A., Foringer, J.R. and Coiffler, B. An integrated clinical approach for the identification, prevention, and treatment of tumor lysis syndrome. Cancer Treatment Reviews. 2010; 36; 164–176.
5. Tosi, P., Barosi, G., Lazzaro,C., Liso,V., Marchetti, M., Morra, E., Pession, A., Rosti, G., Santoro, A., Zinzani, P.L., and Tura, S. Consensus conference on the management of tumor lysis syndrome. Haematologica. 2008; 93(12), 1877–1885

6. Zonfrillo, M.R. Management of pediatric tumor lysis syndrome in the emergency department. Emergency Medical Clinics of North America. 2009; 27; 497–504

7. Holdsworth, M.T. and Nguyen, P. Role of I.V. **Allopurinol** and **Rasburicase** in tumor lysis syndrome. *American Journal of Health-System Pharmacy. 2003; 60(21), 2213–2222*

8. Navolanic, P.M., Pui, C.H., Bishop, M.R., Pearce, T.E., Cairo, M.S., Goldman, S.C., Jeha, S.C., Shanholtz, C.B., Leonard, J.P., and McCubrey, J.A. Elitek- rasburicase: an effective means to prevent and treat hyperuricemia associated with tumor lysis syndrome, a meeting report, Dallas, Texas, January 2002. Leukemia. 2003; 17, 499–514

9. Keneddy, L.D. and Ajiboye, V.O. Rasburicase for the prevention and treatment of hyperuricemia in tumor lysis syndrome. Journal of Oncology Pharmacy Practice. 2010; 16; 205–213

10. Bosly, A., Sonet, A., Pinkerton, C.R., McCowage, G., Bron, D., Sanz, M.A. and Van den Berg, H. Rasburicase (recombinant urate oxidase) for the management of hyperuricemia in patients with cancer: report of an international compassionate use study. Cancer. 2003; 98, 1048–1054

11. Wossmann, W., Schrappe, M., Meyer, U., Zimmermann, M. and Reiter, A. Incidence of tumor lysis syndrome in children with advanced stage Burkitt's lymphoma/leukemia before and after introduction of prophylactic use of urate oxidase. Annals of Hematology. 2003; 82, 160–165

12. Abdullah, S., Diezi, M., Sung, L., Dupuis, L.L., Geary, D. and Abla, O. Sevelamer Hydrochloride: a novel treatment of hyperphosphatemia associated with tumor lysis syndrome in children. Pediatric Blood and Cancer. 2008; 51; 59–61

Chapter 4
Mediastinal Mass and Superior Vena Cava Syndrome

Katrin Scheinemann

Keywords Airway compression • Anesthesia consult • Chest X-ray • Dysphagia • Dyspnea • Echocardiogram • Lymph node biopsy • Mediastinal mass • Right ventricular outflow obstruction • Superior vena cava syndrome

Mediastinal mass can be seen in a variety of childhood cancer: leukemias, lymphomas, neuroblastomas, and rare tumors. Some children are presenting with respiratory symptoms, but a lot of children are surprisingly asymptomatic, and the mass is only picked up on imaging.

A chest X-ray with two views should be taken early in the workup as the result will severely influence the further handling and workup of the patient.

The initial chest X-ray will help to narrow down to differential diagnosis and assess the risk management of the patient.

The mediastinum can be divided into three compartments – the anterior, the middle, and the posterior mediastinum. The anterior mediastinum comprises the thymus gland or its remnants, branches of the internal thoracic artery, and mediastinal lymph nodes. The middle mediastinum contains the pericardium and its contents. The descending aorta, the azygos and hemiazygos vein, the vagus nerve, esophagus, thoracic duct, and some lymph nodes comprise the posterior mediastinum (Fig. 4.1).

Depending on the anatomical structure, certain tumors are characteristic for each compartment.

K. Scheinemann (✉)
Division of Hematology/Oncology, McMaster Children's Hospital,
1200 Main Street West, 555 University Avenue, Hamilton, ON, Canada L8N 3Z5
e-mail: kschein@mcmaster.ca

K. Scheinemann and A.E. Boyce (eds.), *Emergencies in Pediatric Oncology*,
DOI 10.1007/978-1-4614-1174-1_4, © Springer Science+Business Media, LLC 2012

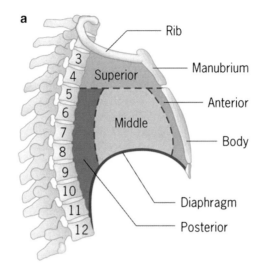

Fig. 4.1 Schematic overview of the mediastinum

Anterior Mediastinum

The most common tumors in the anterior mediastinum can be remembered as the 4 T's:

T-cell lymphoma/leukemia
Teratoma
Thymus
Thyroid malignancy

   Patients with masses in the anterior mediastinum are at high risk for respiratory collapse [1]. Children with respiratory symptoms and an underlying anterior mediastinal mass are at grave risk for total obstruction in the perioperative period. Anesthesia has to be aware for modified handling of these patients to avoid crash intubation or cardiopulmonary resuscitation. Spontaneous ventilation for procedures is preferred in these patients [2].

Middle Mediastinum

The most common tumors in the middle mediastinum are
Lymphoma
Metastatic lesion
Malignant lymphadenopathy

Posterior Mediastinum

The most common tumors in the posterior mediastinum are
Neurogenic tumors (neuroblastoma, pheochromocytoma)
Lymphoma
Ewing's sarcoma
Rhabdomyosarcoma

The anatomical structures of the mediastinum are explaining the expected complications if there is a mass lesion:

Airway compression
Superior vena cava compression
Right ventricular outflow obstruction
Pleural/pericardial effusion
Tumor lysis syndrome

If the initial chest X-ray is showing a mediastinal mass, the immediate handling of the patient has to be adjusted:

Do not lay flat!
Do not sedate!

Often it is the responsibility of the pediatric oncologist to be the messenger of these handling guidelines and supervise them.

Even with the anatomical location of the mediastinal mass, which sometimes is not possible with only an X-ray, further workup investigations are needed:

1. Echocardiogram/ECG should be performed the same day
2. Pulmonary function testing depending on patient's clinical status
3. Anesthesia consultation, if sedation is required for further workup procedures
4. CT neck/chest/abdomen/pelvis if not highly suspicious of leukemia for further staging. It will also help to visualize a possible airway or big vessel compression. It has to be well communicated to everyone that through the CT procedure the patient cannot lay flat
5. Tumor lysis blood work
6. Critical care response team (CCRT)/PICU consult if patient is unstable
7. Careful patient monitoring (cardiac monitor, oxygen saturation)

To finalize the diagnosis, a risk-adapted algorithm is needed as positioning and sedation will increase the risk for these patients. Close communication with anesthesia and surgeons or interventional radiology is needed – every procedure will require careful planning. If the procedure needs to be done awake, patients and parents have to be aware and have to be guided through it.

A stepwise approach could look like this – it will start from the least invasive procedure:

1. CBC – if no peripheral blasts or high enough white cell count – not diagnostic

2. BMA/BMBx – needs to be possibly done without sedation and different positioning – will sometimes require anterior access [please see Chap. 9 for further details]
3. Tap of pleural/pericardial effusion possible – not the best diagnostic tool
4. Lymph node biopsy if peripheral lymphadenopathy – no core biopsy, lymph node removal needed for accurate diagnosis
5. Biopsy mediastinal mass either through interventional radiology or surgery

The use of steroids to shrink the mediastinal mass should be avoided as much as possible for proper diagnosis. If patient is unstable, discussion with PICU and anesthesia has to take place about the timing of starting steroids and the procedure.

Treatment should be initiated as soon as possible to decrease morbidity.

Superior Vena Cava Syndrome (SVCS)

The syndrome occurs in case of a compression of the vessel either internally or externally (Fig. 4.2). Major cause for an internal compression would be a blood clot caused by an indwelling venous catheter; major cause for an external compression is lymphadenopathy. It is much more common in the adult world especially seen in lung cancer patients [3].

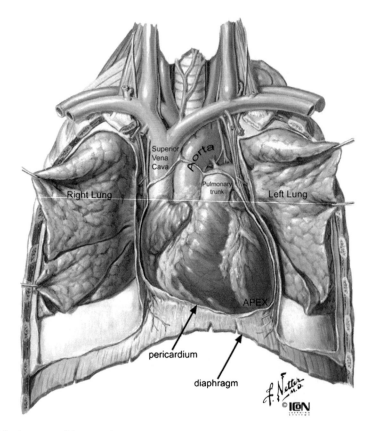

Fig. 4.2 Anatomy of the superior vena cava

Symptoms of SVCS are [4]:

1. Nonproductive cough
2. Dyspnea
3. Dysphagia
4. Hoarseness
5. Chest pain
6. Edema of the face/neck or peripheral
7. Prominent venous pattern

Imaging studies including chest X-ray or CT, ultrasound, or echocardiogram should be performed according to the planned further workup.

Similar to patients with a mediastinal mass, positioning is one of the most important treatments – do not lay the patient flat. Oxygen treatment can also be beneficial.

The role of high dose steroids for lymphadenopathy is controversial – a diagnosis has to be established prior to initiation of steroids.

Treatment for the underlying cause should be initiated as soon as possible.

Case 1

An 8-year-old boy presented with a 1-month history of shortness of breath, cough, and chest pain. Clinical examination revealed lymphadenopathy on the left side of the neck. Lymph node biopsy and bone marrow biopsies were done under local anesthesia; diagnosis of T-cell lymphoblastic lymphoma was confirmed (Fig. 4.3).

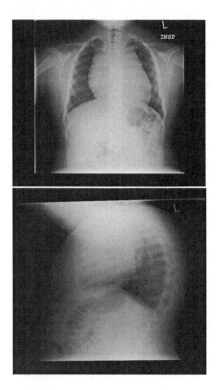

Fig. 4.3 Large anterior mediastinal mass noted. Trachea is displaced

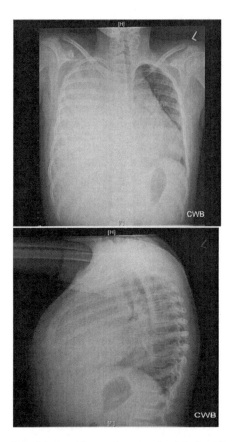

Fig. 4.4 Opacification of the right hemithroax obscuring the right hemidiaphragm. Shifting of the mediastinum and the heart to the left side

Case 2

A 12-year-old boy presented with a 3-month history of progressive weight loss, shortness of breath, orthopnea, and cough. Clinical examination revealed splenomegaly, severe orthopnea (sleep at 45° angle), and decreased air entry in the right side. Diagnosis of a T-cell ALL was made (Fig. 4.4).

References

1. Ben-Ari J, Schonfeld T, Harlev E, Steinberg R, Yaniv I, Katz J, Schwartz M, Freud E. Life-threatening airway obstruction secondary to mass in children – a preventable event? Pediatric Emergency Care 2005; 21 (7): 427–430
2. Stricker PA, Gurnaney HG, Litman RS. Anesthetic management of children with an anterior mediastinal mass. Journal of clinical anesthesia 2010; 22: 159–163
3. Walji N, Chan AK, Peake DR. Common acute oncological emergencies: diagnosis, investigation and management. Postgrad Med J 2008; 84: 418–427
4. Colen FN. Oncologic emergencies: superior vena cava syndrome, tumor lysis syndrome, and spinal cord compression. J Emerg Nurs 2008; 34 (6): 535–537

Chapter 5
Abdominal Masses

Katrin Scheinemann

Keywords Abdominal compartment syndrome • Abdominal masses • Ultrasound • Decompression • Intra-abdominal hypertension • Intra-abdominal hypertension

Many childhood malignancies are localized in the abdomen. Wilms' tumor, neuroblastoma, and germ cell tumors can often grow to an enormous size before the children will become symptomatic. It seems that compensation is possible over a long period of time, but once the children become symptomatic, they can decompensate very quickly, and immediate intervention is necessary.

The intra-abdominal pressure is defined as steady-state pressure concealed within the abdominal cavity [1]. Normal value is around 0 mmHg. It increases with inspiration and decreases with expiration due to diaphragmatic contraction and relaxation. Intra-abdominal hypertension can then lead to an abdominal compartment syndrome which leads to end-organ dysfunction and will require immediate intervention.

Risk factors within pediatric oncology include [2]:

1. Massive fluid resuscitation for septic shock
2. Pancreatitis
3. Intra-abdominal tumors
4. Ileus
5. Mechanical ventilation
6. Postoperative complications like hemorrhage

K. Scheinemann (✉)
Division of Hematology/Oncology, McMaster Children's Hospital,
1200 Main Street West, 555 University Avenue, Hamilton, ON, Canada L8N 3Z5
e-mail: kschein@mcmaster.ca

K. Scheinemann and A.E. Boyce (eds.), *Emergencies in Pediatric Oncology*, DOI 10.1007/978-1-4614-1174-1_5, © Springer Science+Business Media, LLC 2012

An abdominal compartment syndrome will also affect other organ systems [3]:

1. Respiratory (elevation of diaphragm leads to increased intrathoracic pressure)
2. Cardiovascular (compression on the inferior vena cava and portal vein leads to reduced venous return)
3. Renal (direct compression of renal vessel or decreased cardiac output)
4. Gastrointestinal (decreased perfusion leads to mucosal ischemia)
5. Hepatic (decreased perfusion leads to tissue hypoxia and coagulopathy)
6. Central nervous system (elevated intracranial pressure)

The best intervention is prevention to minimize the morbidity. Early recognition and anticipation is the most important tool. The longer the hypertension is unrecognized, the higher the morbidity and mortality.

The following diagnostic tools can be helpful in the assessment of intra-abdominal hypertension:

1. Abdominal exam including abdominal girth measurement

   • Distension
   • Organomegaly
   • Mass/tumor palpable (very careful palpation – risk of tumor rupture!)
   • Bowel sounds
   • Prominent surface vein pattern
   • Swelling of lower limbs and/or scrotum

2. Abdominal US including Doppler:

   • Masses
   • Organ size and vessel flow
   • Ascites/pleural effusion
   • Bowel wall thickness
   • Lymph nodes

3. Urinary output/bowel movements (stool to be tested for occult blood)
4. Chest X-ray two views
5. Bloodwork: BGA, electrolytes, liver and renal function testing, coagulation screen
6. Echocardiogram

All of the above-mentioned tools can be done at bedside, so patient does not need to be moved.

The management includes regular monitoring and optimizing systemic perfusion and organ function, but whenever feasible, decompression should be achieved.

Medical treatment could include:

1. Body positioning (head elevation)
2. Drainage via NG tube
3. Fluid resuscitation to maintain hemodynamics
4. Diuretics and continuous renal replacement therapy

Acute decompression is sometimes necessary if the medical treatment is not sufficient enough and the patient is developing multiorgan failure. The following treatment modalities are available for acute to subacute decompression:

1. Percutaneous catheter decompression
2. Surgical abdominal decompression
3. Emergency radiation (see Chap. 16 for more details)

Even with acute decompression, continuous medical treatment and monitoring are still warranted as long-term morbidity is high. Early implementation of chemotherapy should also be considered but will not release pressure as quickly, and dosing has to be adjusted due to possible renal, liver, and cardiac impairment.

Case 1

A 4-year-old boy presented with a 10-day history of progressive abdominal pain and bed-wetting. Clinical exam revealed a distended abdomen and tenderness over the left flank with impression of a mass. Bloodwork was normal. A CT revealed a large mass arising from the left kidney. Patient was taken to the OR for tumor removal without intraoperative rupture. Pathology confirmed diagnosis of Wilms' tumor (Fig. 5.1).

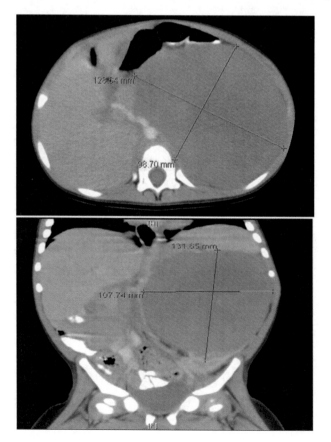

Fig. 5.1 Abdominal CT

Case 2

An 11-year-old girl presented with a 1-day history of abdominal distension and pain. Clinical exam revealed only a firm abdominal mass; blood work was unremarkable. A CT showed a huge mass most likely arising from the adnexa. Patient was taken to the OR within a day, and a gross total resection, including salpingo-oophorectomy, was achieved. Pathology revealed a malignant germ cell tumor (Fig. 5.2).

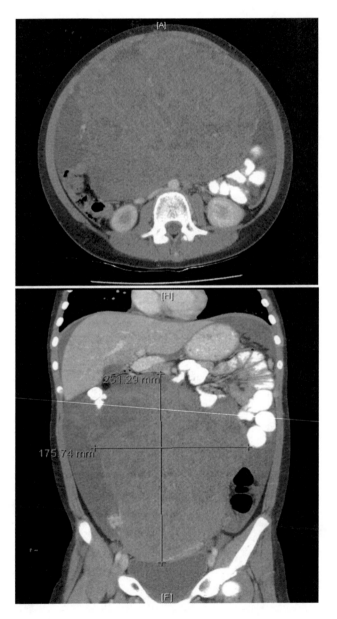

Fig. 5.2 Abdominal CT

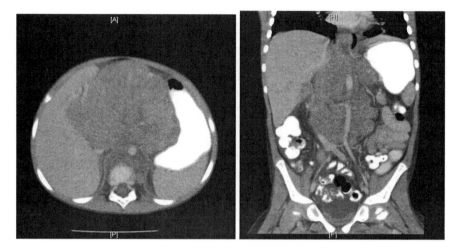

Fig. 5.3 Abdominal CT

Case 3

A 3.5-year-old girl presented with a 2-week history of abdominal pain, but abdominal distension for only one day. Urgent CT scan revealed a large soft tissue mesenteric mass with encasement of renal arteries, extensive lymphadenopathy, as well as bilateral pleural effusion. Biopsy and further investigation revealed stage IV neuroblastoma. Patient experienced renal impairment and hypoalbuminemia after initiation of treatment (chemotherapy). Surgical intervention was not necessary.

First resection attempt had to be stopped due to massive bleeding, and abdominal cavity was not closed by the end of procedure (bleeding control and packing). Patient had massive abdominal compartment syndrome with ARDS, hemorrhagic shock, DIC, pleural effusion, and acute renal failure. After recovery, a second surgical attempt led to 20% debulking which was well tolerated (Fig. 5.3).

References

1. Malbrain MLNG, Vidts W, Ravyts M, de Laet I, de Waele J. Acute intestinal distress syndrome: the importance of intra-abdominal pressure. Minverva Anestesiology 2008; 74: 657–673
2. Carlotti APCP, Carvalho WB. Abdominal compartment syndrome. A review. Pediatric Critical Care Medicine 2009; 10 (1): 115–120
3. Kawar B, Siplovich L. Abdominal compartment syndrome in children: the dilemma of treatment. European Journal of Pediatric Surgery 2003; 13: 330–333

Chapter 6
Spinal Cord Compression and Cauda Equina Syndrome

Katrin Scheinemann

Keywords Cauda equina syndrome • Constipation • High-dose steroids • Motor weakness • Sciatica • Spinal cord compression • Urinary retention

Spinal cord compression or cauda equina syndrome is a frequent complication in pediatric malignancies. Quite often, it is one of the presenting symptoms – varying from a sudden onset to a more chronic pattern. On estimation, between 4 and 25% of all children diagnosed with cancer will develop SCC or CES [1]. Sometimes, SCC or CES occurs throughout treatment, either as new metastatic disease or as treatment complication, e.g., bleeding or myelitis following intrathecal chemotherapy [2].

As this is a neurologic emergency, urgent diagnosis and treatment is warranted. Suspicion should be raised with the following symptoms [3].

Early clinical symptoms of SCC are:

1. Urinary retention
2. Constipation
3. Urinary incontinence
4. Fecal incontinence
5. Back pain

Back pain is described as the earliest symptom lasting for quite some time prior to diagnosis [4]. Due to the age group, it can be quite unspecific in children, and they may complain of "tummy pain" instead of back pain. Pain associated with positioning (walking vs. sitting vs. lying down) or coughing and sneezing should be further investigated.

K. Scheinemann (✉)
Division of Hematology/Oncology, McMaster Children's Hospital,
1200 Main Street West, 555 University Avenue, Hamilton, ON, Canada L8N 3Z5
e-mail: kschein@mcmaster.ca

K. Scheinemann and A.E. Boyce (eds.), *Emergencies in Pediatric Oncology*,
DOI 10.1007/978-1-4614-1174-1_6, © Springer Science+Business Media, LLC 2012

Late clinical symptoms of SCC are:

1. Motor weakness
2. Sensory impairment
3. Sensory loss
4. Paralysis

The younger the children are, the more difficult the assessment of these symptoms will be, especially if they have not been toilet trained or are not walking yet. Also, sensory impairment or loss is quite difficult to figure out as younger children will not have verbal skills to do so. Instead, the anal sphincter tone or cremasteric reflex can be tested.

Clinical symptoms of CES are:

1. Low back pain
2. Unilateral or bilateral sciatica
3. Motor weakness of lower extremities
4. Sensory disturbance in saddle area
5. Loss of visceral function

It is very important to do a thorough neurological exam and document the findings, including the estimated level and the timeline, as this will determine progression/recovery potential.

Imaging of choice is MRI of spine and pelvis. In cases of concerns for bony involvement, a CT may be needed.

In a large series from Argentina, the most common underlying tumors were localized extradural and included sarcomas (rhabdomyosarcoma and Ewing's sarcoma) and neuroblastomas [1]. Other entities include primary CNS tumors and metastatic spread from leukemias.

If imaging is confirming an intraspinal mass with acute symptoms, neurosurgery should be contacted for a possible decompression and tumor sampling. The early start of high-dose steroids is helpful to reduce the swelling, but please keep in mind that the diagnosis (e.g., leukemic infiltrate or lymphoma) can be altered or made impossible by this. High-dose steroids seemed to improve the outcome/neurological recovery despite the side effects [5]. Tapering should be started as early as possible to minimize side effects.

If surgery is not an option, radiation oncology should be contacted (please see Chapter 16 for further information).

If neither surgical intervention nor radiation seems feasible, chemotherapy should be initiated as soon as possible. Especially in tumors like neuroblastoma, this seems to be beneficial [6].

The degree of aggressive intervention depends on the length of symptoms – paraparesis/paraplegia lasting for over 48 h has a low potential for recovery. Motor dysfunction has a better potential for recovery compared to neurologic bladder or bowel dysfunction.

Even with immediate relief of the pressure, neurological recovery will take some time and additional care needs to be taken:

1. Pain control – As medications for neuropathic pain need to be titrated, acute pain medications should be initiated first
2. Urinary retention – One time catheterization or insertion of a Foley catheter
3. Urinary incontinence – Watch out for urinary infection; antibiotic prophylaxis should be discussed
4. Constipation – Should be treated aggressively as increased risk of ileus and infection
5. Early initiation of physiotherapy and occupational therapy for paresis

Urology and pain service should be consulted early to help with the management. Also, some centers have specialist for spinal cord injury rehabilitation which can be of great help.

Case 1

An 8-month-old boy was referred to ER for a 1-month history of irritability and increasing weakness of his lower extremities. Clinical exam revealed significant weakness in both lower limbs with only some toe movement and areflexia. Patient underwent urgent MRI spine which revealed extradural mass from T-12 to L-3. He was taken to the OR immediately for decompressive surgery and was started on high-dose steroids. Pathology revealed to be neuroblastoma. Patient underwent complete recovery from his neurological symptoms (Fig. 6.1).

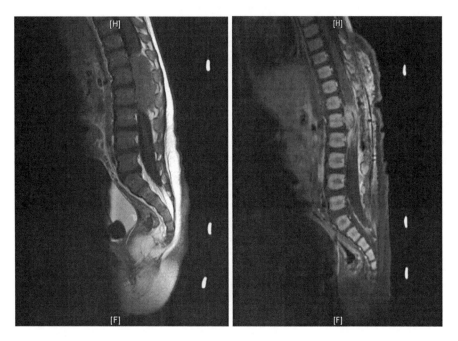

Fig. 6.1 Sagittal MRI pre-(*left*) and post-operative (*right*)

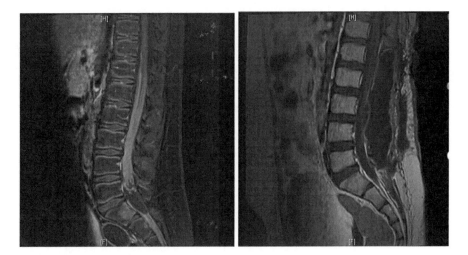

Fig. 6.2 Sagittal MRI pre-(*left*) and post-operative (*right*)

Case 2

An 11-year-old boy with a previous history of acute lymphoblastic leukemia (ALL) 7 years ago presented with a 6-week history of progressive back pain radiating into his buttocks and thighs and leg weakness. He was unable to ambulate for 4 weeks prior to his admission. Also, at least three incidents of urine incontinence were recorded. Clinical exam revealed significant muscle weakness of his lower extremities with hyperalgesia in his buttocks.

MRI revealed a sacral mass with thickening of his cauda equina. He was immediately started on high-dose steroids and was taken to the OR for decompressive surgery. Further investigation revealed relapse of his ALL. Neurologically, he is able to walk again with a walker, no bladder or bowel dysfunction, and no sensory dysfunction (Fig. 6.2).

Case 3

A 15-year-old girl presented with a 2-year history of chronic back pain radiating into her legs. She also described numbness below her knee for almost 9 months, with no hyperesthesia sensation.

MRI revealed extensive syringohydromegaly from the medullary junction down to conus medullaris. There was also an enhancing mass with cystic areas extending from T-9 to T-12. She was taken to the OR for a 5 level laminectomy and tumor resection which was achieved a near total tumor resection. Postoperatively, her motor function recovered, but she developed a neurogenic bladder which still requires intermittent catheterization.

Pathology revealed the diagnosis of a WHO II ependymoma (Fig. 6.3).

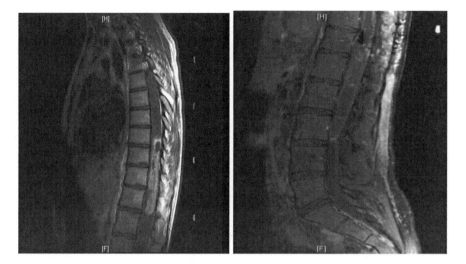

Fig. 6.3   Sagittal MRI pre-(*left*) and post-operative (*right*)

References

1. Pollono D, Tomarchia S, Drut R, Ibanez O, Ferreyra M, Cedola J. Spinal cord compression: a review of 70 patients. Pediatric Hematology and Oncology 2003; 20: 457–466
2. Amini A, Liu JK, Kan P, Brockmeyer DL. Cerebrospinal fluid dissecting into spinal epidural space after lumbar puncture causing cauda equina syndrome: review of literature and illustrative case. Childs Nerv Syst 2006; 22: 1639–1641
3. Colen FN. Oncologic emergencies: superior vena cava syndrome, tumor lysis syndrome, and spinal cord compression. Journal of emergency nursing 2008; 34: 535–537
4. Walji N, Chan AK, Peake DR. Common acute oncological emergencies: diagnosis, investigation and management. Postgrad Med J 2008; 84: 418–427
5. Yalamanchili M, Lesser GJ. Malignant spinal cord compression. Current treatment options in oncology 2003; 4: 509–516
6. Walter KN, Kratz C, Uhl M, Niemeyer C. Chemotherapy as a therapeutic option for congenital neuroblastoma complicated by paraplegia. Klinische Paediatrie 2008; 20: 175–177

Chapter 7
Fever and Neutropenia

Stephanie Cox

Keywords Aminoglycoside • Antibiotics • Bone marrow recovery • Central venous catheters • Fever • Gram-negative • Gram-positive bacteria • Inflammatory signs • Neutropenia • Oral mucosa • Prophylactic antibiotics • Respiratory distress • Sepsis • Septic emboli • Tunnel infection • β-lactam antibiotic

Overview

Intensive cytotoxic chemotherapy regimens that often cause profound neutropenia place the child undergoing treatment for cancer at risk for life-threatening infection. Fever and neutropenia in children with malignancy carries a mortality rate of 1% and imposes significant morbidity upon patients and the families supporting those patients [1]. Fever is often the only sign of potentially life-threatening infection, and the rates of sepsis among children with cancer age 1–9 years is 12.8% and age 10–19 years is 17.4% [2]. Due to the serious nature of this consequence of therapy, this chapter focuses on the rapid recognition, assessment, evaluation, and treatment of the pediatric patient with fever and neutropenia.

Definitions

Fever – A single oral temperature of ≥ 38.3°C or a temperature of ≥38°C for ≥ 1 h continuously or at two times with a minimum interval of 12 h [2–5]. Measuring the temperature orally is the preferred route; however, if the pediatric patient is unable

S. Cox (✉)
Division of Hematology/Oncology, McMaster Children's Hospital
1280 Main Street West, Hamilton, ON, Canada L8S 4K1
e-mail: coxst@hhsc.ca

K. Scheinemann and A.E. Boyce (eds.), *Emergencies in Pediatric Oncology*,
DOI 10.1007/978-1-4614-1174-1_7, © Springer Science+Business Media, LLC 2012

to use an oral thermometer, axillary measurement is acceptable. Conservative guidelines suggest adding 0.3°C to 0.5°C the axillary temperatures [5]. An axillary temperature of 37.8°C is considered a fever. Rectal temperatures are to be avoided in the neutropenic patient due to concerns of mucosal trauma and bacteremia. Fever is often the sole sign of infection in the neutropenic host; however, infection must be considered if any signs of clinical deterioration are present regardless of temperature [4, 5].

Neutropenia – A neutrophil count of <500 cells/mm^3 or a count of <1,000 cells/mm^3 with a predicted decline to <500 cells/mm^3 within 48 h [2, 3]. The risk of infection is greatest at a neutrophil count of ≤100 cells/mm^3 [2, 5].

Sepsis – Systemic inflammatory response syndrome (temperature >38.5°C or <36.0°C, tachycardia >2 SD for age or bradycardia if <1 year, respiratory rate >2 SD for age, white blood cells above or below age norms not related to chemotherapy) in the presence of proven or suspected infection [6].

Septic shock – Sepsis plus cardiovascular dysfunction (hypotension, vasopressor dependence, acidosis, elevated lactate, oliguria, delayed capillary refill, core to peripheral temperature gap >3°C) [6].

Etiology

The epidemiology of neutropenic infections varies within treatment centers and only 10–30% of neutropenic fevers will have an identified microbiologic source [6]. Thus, the majority of febrile neutropenic episodes will be treated as a fever of indeterminate origin. It is important to note that there can be noninfectious causes of fever in this population including certain chemotherapy agents such as cytarabine and hematologic malignancy. When there is a positive microbiologic source, 85–90% are either gram-positive or gram-negative bacteria [6]. Gram-positive bacteria are responsible for up to 60–70% of microbiologically confirmed cases of fever and neutropenia [3].

Most common potential infectious etiologies in febrile neutropenic children include [3, 6]:

1. *Bacterial* – Gram positive: *Staphylococcus* spp*, *Streptococcus* spp*, *Enterococcus* spp* *Corynebacterium* spp*, *Bacillus* spp, *Clostridium* spp
   Gram negative: *Escherichia coli**, *Pseudomonas aeruginosa**, *Klebsiella* spp*, *Enterobacter* spp, anaerobes
   *The most common causes of bacteremia
2. *Viral* – Herpes simplex, varicella zoster, respiratory syncytial virus, influenza A and B, parainfluenza, adenovirus, rotavirus, enterovirus, cytomegalovirus, epstein-barr, human herpes virus 6, BK virus, JC virus
3. *Fungal* – *Candida* spp, *Aspergillus* spp, Zygomycetes, *Fusarium* spp, *Scedosporium* spp, *Cryptococcus neoformans*
4. *Other* – *Pneumocystis jiroveci*, protozoa, chemotherapy-related fever

Risk Factors

The standard of care for pediatric oncology patients with fever and neutropenia is to receive parental antibiotics in a hospital care setting. There has been an effort to assess the risk factors in this population that may make them suitable for outpatient management. Some of the identified factors include:

1. *Low Risk* – temperature <39°C, monocyte count ≥1,000 cells/mm^3, lack of medical comorbidity, lack of radiographic evidence of pneumonia, outpatient status at time of febrile episode, anticipated duration of neutropenia ≤5 days, malignancy other than acute myelogenous leukemia
2. *High Risk* – Duration of neutropenia ≥10 days, <7 days between last chemotherapy and onset of fever, pneumonitis, severe mucositis, signs of compensated or decompensated shock, dehydration, hypotension, respiratory distress or compromise, failure of major organ system, relapsed leukemia, treatment with high-dose cytarabine, less than 1 year of age, C-reactive protein >90 mg/L, platelet count <50, and neutrophils <100 cells/mm^3, serum polymerase chain reaction ≥90 mg/L

Assessment and Evaluation

The assessment and evaluation of the pediatric patient with fever and neutropenia requires a systematic approach paying particular attention to the unique characteristics of this population.

History – A full pediatric history should be taken but particular detail to try to identify source of infection and the risk of sepsis should be gathered including:

- Type of malignancy
- Treatment regimen including details of the most recent therapy received
- Fever including maximum and duration and associated chills, shaking, or rigors
- Current symptoms including orthostatic symptoms, myalgias, headache, cough, rhinorrhea, shortness of breath, chest pain, ear pain, sore throat, abdominal pain, vomiting, diarrhea, pain with urination, and skin lesions
- Oral intake including nausea and vomiting and stool history
- Potential exposures including home and school contacts
- Review all current medications including colony-stimulating factors and compliance with prophylactic antibiotics
- History of previous febrile infections

Vital Signs – A full set of vital signs should be obtained and reassessed every 30 to 60 minutes until the patient is stable and should include:

- Temperature – maximum, duration, frequency, and responsiveness to antipyretic medication is useful in assessing risk of sepsis.

- Respiratory rate – tachypnea and increased work of breathing can be early signs of sepsis.
- Heart rate – tachycardia when out of proportion with fever, crying, pain, or anxiety should be considered compensatory shock.
- Blood pressure – hypotension should be considered a late sign of impending septic shock.
- Pulse oximetry – hypoxia may represent pneumonitis or evolving consolidation.
- Weight – useful in assessing degree of dehydration.

Physical Exam – A quick assessment of the child's severity of illness should include the patient's color, muscle tone, degree of activity, respiratory pattern, mental status, skin temperature, pulses, and capillary refill [6]. Classic inflammatory signs of infection including temperature, edema, erythema, and suppuration may be reduced secondary to the impaired immune system. Pay particular attention to the following sites as often the presence of discrete to moderate pain may be the only indicator of infection [2]:

- Eyes and sinuses
- Oral mucosa – including the moisture of mucous membranes and presence, characteristics, and extent of mucositis
- Lungs – assessing work of breathing and auscultated for air entry including the presence of cough, wheeze, or crackles
- Cardiovascular assessment – including color and temperature of the skin, quality of pulses, and time of capillary refill
- Abdomen – including the quality of bowel sounds, assessing for tenderness, and presence of hepatosplenomegaly
- The perineum – including genital and anal areas assessing for rash, discharge, fissures, hemorrhoids, or lesions
- Skin – including folds, sites of vascular access catheters, bone marrow and lumbar puncture sites, and tissue around nails looking for erythema, warmth, tenderness, or fluctuance
- Site of surgery – when present, assessing the incision sites for discharge and the quality and state of healing

Diagnostic Evaluation

Diagnostic testing and evaluation should focus on determining the etiology of the infectious agent and be individualized based on the findings on the history and physical exam (Table 7.1).

Table 7.1 Investigations and evaluations for patients with F/N

Test	Indication	Special Considerations
Complete blood count with manual differential	For all patients to assess degree of neutropenia, anemia, and thrombocytopenia	Degree of myelosuppression is an important risk factor for sepsis
Creatinine, urea, electrolytes, transaminases	For all patients to assess for excessive fluid losses and plan for supportive care and monitor for drug toxicity	Should be reassessed every 3 days or more frequently based on therapy regimen and patient status
Amylase, lipase	For patients with signs and symptoms consistent with pancreatitis	Recent therapy with asparaginase is a risk factor
Blood culture	For all patients who present with fever	Draw from each lumen of a central venous catheter and peripheral vein. Bacterial growth found in CVL sample 2 h or more before other sample suggests CVL as site of infection. Repeat samples for patients with positive samples or persistent fever is indicated
Urine culture	In patients with urinary symptoms or neoplasms in urinary or renal areas	Classic indicators for urinary tract infection including urinalysis positive for white blood cells, nitrites, or blood may not be present. Culture urine regardless of urinalysis if high index of suspicion as site of infection. Assessing for virology in post hematopoietic stem cell patients with hematuria may be indicated
Stool cultures	In patients with diarrhea or abdominal pain	Include testing for culture and sensitivity, virology, and *C. difficile* in all patients. Assessing for ova and parasites can be done on patients with risk factors or symptoms
Culture of lesions or wounds	In patients with any vesicular lesions, erythema, or exudate	Any rash suspected of VZV or HSV should be swabbed. Pay particular attention to central venous catheter sites, bone marrow biopsy sites, lumbar puncture sites, and surgical sites
Oral swabs	In patients with evidence of mucositis, oral lesions or white plaques on hard palette, or buccal mucosa	Swabs for both mycology and virology are indicated in patients with mucositis. Throat culture for patients suspected group A streptococcus

(continued)

Table 7.1 (continued)

Test	Indication	Special Considerations
Nasopharyngeal swab	In patients with upper respiratory tract infection symptoms or exposure to influenza A, B, or RSV	Contraindicated in patients with thrombocytopenia with a platelet count <20, may require transfusion prior to obtaining sample
Culture of cerebral spinal fluid	In patients with suspected CNS infection or meningeal signs	Contraindicated in patients with a platelet count <50, require transfusion prior to obtaining sample
Chest radiograph (2 views)	In patients with respiratory abnormalities	Incidence of pneumonia on CXR in febrile neutropenic patients 3–6% with almost all being associated with clinical signs and symptoms[5]
Abdominal Radiograph	In patients with focal abdominal tenderness or suspected typhlitis	Images need to be interpreted in the context of the profoundly neutropenic patient
Ultrasound	In patients with focal abdominal tenderness, suspected typhlitis, suspected surgical abdomen, or other suspected infection in the soft tissues	Images need to be interpreted in the context of the profoundly neutropenic patient
Echocardiogram	In patients with positive bacterial cultures associated with cardiac vegetations or in patients with persistent fevers with associated CVL dysfunction/clots	Although more invasive transesophageal echo is more sensitive than transthoracic studies for detecting cardiac vegetations
CT scan	In patients with persistent fevers and suspected fungal infections, suspected typhlitis, or abscess formation	Images need to be interpreted in the context of the profoundly neutropenic patient
MRI scan	In patients with suspected CNS infections or bony source of infection	Images need to be interpreted in the context of the profoundly neutropenic patient

Treatment

As the progression of infection in the febrile pediatric oncology patient can be rapid, the benefit of early initiation of empiric antimicrobial therapy in decreasing morbidity and mortality is well established. The cornerstone of therapy in this population is broad-spectrum empiric parenteral antibiotics that are effective against gram-positive and gram-negative organisms most likely to cause illness in this population. The goal of antimicrobial therapy is to be effective against a wide range of potential pathogens. An important note is that clinicians should evaluate neutropenic patients who are unwell but afebrile and nonneutropenic patients who are febrile and expected to become neutropenic. These patients should be treated as per fever and neutropenia therapy on a clinical basis [1].

Antimicrobial Therapy

The antibiotic regimen used should be institutional specific, taking into consideration the type, frequency of occurrence, and antibiotic susceptibility of bacterial isolates identified at the hospital.

General principles of empiric therapy include the use of:

- Combination therapy – β-lactam antibiotic plus an aminoglycoside. Benefits include synergistic effects against pathogens and possible reduction in emergence of antibiotic resistant organisms. Disadvantages include the toxicity, particularly nephro- and ototoxicity of the aminoglycosides.
- Monotherapy – broad-spectrum β-lactam antibiotic with antipseudomonal activity. Many centers now use monotherapy as standard therapy for episodes of uncomplicated fever and neutropenia as there is evidence that it is as efficacious as combination therapy [5].

Additional coverage may be warranted including the addition of:

- Vancomycin – for patients with hypotension or other cardiopulmonary deterioration, who have received high-dose cytarabine due to increased risk of alpha hemolytic streptococcus infections, substantial mucositis, clinical suspicion of CVC infection, or in patients with history of MRSA or recent exposure
- Triple therapy – including metronidazole, 3rd or 4th generation cephalosporin, and vancomycin for patients with a clinical suspicion of typhlitis, abdominal pain, or blood from the rectum who require better anaerobic activity of therapy

Indications for therapy modifications include [5]:

- Change in clinical status or vital signs, unstable patient, or worsening of symptoms and signs: change antibiotics
- Persistent fever during first 3–5 days of treatment:
  If no change: continue antibiotics, discontinue vancomycin if cultures negative
  If progressive disease: change antibiotics
- Persistent fever greater than 5 days: consider adding an antifungal drug with or without antibiotic changes
- Identification of pathogen: adjust antibiotics to most appropriate treatment
- Development of signs and symptoms of a localized infection: adjust antibiotics to most appropriate treatment

Indications for Central Venous Catheter Removal

Central venous catheters (CVC) have become essential in the administration of chemotherapy and in the supportive care of pediatric oncology patients but are a potential source of infection. The removal of the CVC may be required under the following
circumstances [3]:

- Recurrent infection
- Response to antibiotic not apparent after 2–3 days
- Evidence of tunnel infection
- Evidence of periport infection
- Septic emboli
- Hypotension associated with catheter use
- Nonpatent catheter
- Bacteremia due to *Bacillus* sp., *P.* aeruginosa, *Stenotrophomonas maltophilia*,
  C. jeikeium, VRE, *Acinetobater*
- Fungemia secondary to *Candida* sp.

Duration of Therapy

The course of antimicrobial therapy required by patients should be reassessed after
48–72 h. Decision to continue, step up, step down, or discontinue antimicrobial
therapy needs to be individualized based on patient presentation, risk factors,
response to therapy, and identification of pathogen. Often, the complicated febrile
and neutropenic pediatric patient warrants a consult with the infectious disease service for ongoing management. Bacteremic episodes require a treatment course of a
minimum of 7–14 days and individualized as per the culture and sensitivity of the
identified pathogen [5].

Guidelines for the duration of antibiotics include [5]:

- All patients are to receive a minimum of 48 h of empiric therapy then
- Afebrile on day 3 and patient is:

  Afebrile for 24–48 h
  No identified source of fever
  Sterile blood cultures
  Evidence of bone marrow recovery defined as sustained increase in platelet count
      and absolute neutrophil or absolute phagocyte count

  → Stop antibiotic therapy
- If no evidence of bone marrow recovery and patient is for:

  → Low risk: continue antibiotics until patient is afebrile 5–7 days
  → High risk: continue antibiotics until recovery of neutrophil count and patient
      is well

- Persistent fever on day three and patient has:

  Absolute neutrophil count ≥500/μL
  Continue antibiotics until 4 of 5 days after absolute neutrophil count ≥500/μL, then reassess
  Absolute neutrophil count <500/μL
  Continue antibiotics for 2 more weeks, reassess, and stop if no disease sites found

Case 1

A 13-year-old boy treated for AML developed prolonged fever and neutropenia post cycle 4 of his treatment. CT chest reveals right upper lobe airspace disease highly suggestive of invasive aspergillosis. Antifungal treatment initiated (Fig. 7.1).

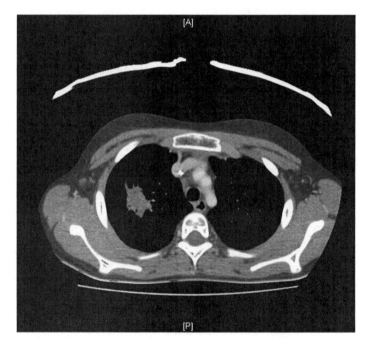

Fig. 7.1 CT image with mass like focal area of airspace disease in the apical segment of the right upper lobe surrounded by a halo of groundglass opacity

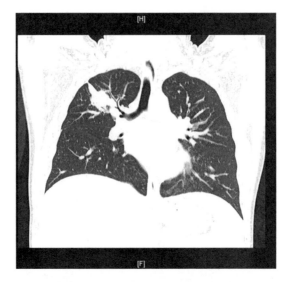

Fig. 7.1 (continued)

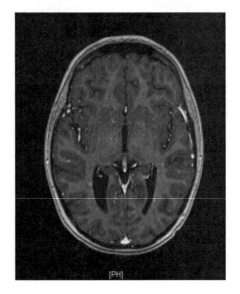

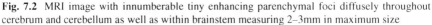

Fig. 7.2 MRI image with innumberable tiny enhancing parenchymal foci diffusely throughout cerebrum and cerebellum as well as within brainstem measuring 2–3mm in maximum size

Case 2

A 13-year-old girl with underlying diagnosis of AML Multiple febrile neutropenia episodes with *Streptococcus mitis* requiring multiple central line changes. Post cycle 4, she developed severe headache and eye symptoms including blurred vision, scleral erythema and pain. MRI head revealed innumerable tiny enhancing lesions scattered throughout her brain parenchyma highly suggestive for septic emboli. Prolonged course of antibiotics and antifugal treatment until complete remission (Fig. 7.2).

References

1. Chamberlain, J., Smibert, E., Skeen, J., Alvaro, F. Prospective audit of treatment of paediatric febrile neutropenia in Australiasia. J. paediatr. Child Health. 2005; 41: 598–603.
2. Mendes, A., Sapolnik, R., Mendonca, N. New guidelines for the clinical management of febrile neutropenia and sepsis in pediatric oncology patients. Jornal de Pediatria. 2007; 83(2)S54.
3. Hughes, W., Armstrong, D., Bodey, G., Bow, E., Brown, A., et al. 2002 Guidelines for the Use of Antimicrobial Agents in Neutropenic Patients with Cancer. CID. 2002; 34: 730–751.
4. Larson, R. Prophylaxis of infection during chemotherapy-induced neutropenia. In: UpToDate, Drews, R (Ed), UpToDate, Waltham, MA, 2010.
5. Bertuch, A. Fever in children with chemotherapy-induced neutropenia. In: UpToDate, Edwards, M., Poplack, D. (Eds), Waltham, MA, 2010.
6. Meckler, G., Lindemulder, S. Fever and Neutropenia in Pediatric Patients with Cancer. Emergency Medicine Clinics of North America. 2009; 27(3).
7. Fleischhack, G., Schmidt-Niemann, M., Wulff, B., Havers, W., Marklein, G., et al. Piperacillin, beta-lactam inhibitor plus gentamicin as empirical therapy of a sequential regimen in febrile neutropenia of pediatric cancer patients. Support Care Cancer. 2001; 9: 372–279.
8. Lex, C., Korholz, D., Kohlmuller, B., Bonig, H., Willers, R., et al. Infectious complications in children with acute lymphoblastic leukemia and T-cell lymphoma-a rational for tailored supportive care. Support Care Cancer. 2001; 9: 514–521.

Chapter 8
Procedures

Katrin Scheinemann

Keywords Bone marrow aspiration • Conscious sedation • Dry tap • Local anesthetic • Lumbar puncture • Trendelenburg

Conscious sedation for lumbar puncture and bone marrow aspiration and biopsy has become available in 1991, but is not used in all centers. However, no one would disagree that this has improved the quality of life for patients and caregivers quite a lot.

Lumbar puncture and intrathecal chemotherapy.

Lumbar punctures can be performed either in a sitting position or lying on the site – depending on the performing physician's experience.

It is necessary to ensure that patients/parents have consented to the procedure. The main risks are postprocedure low-pressure headache and nausea, infection, or neurological complications.

The most important point of performing a lumbar puncture is positioning. Patients should be placed in the left or right (depending on performing person's dexterity) lateral position. They should be lying on a hard surface. Their neck and knees should be bent in full flexion – the goal is a fetal position. The area should then be prepped in an aseptic technique. Palpate the iliac crest on both sites – this is approximately the level of L 4/5. Go one level below – just in case you will get a bloody tap and have to go for another level. The needle should be inserted in a 90-degree angle from the spine. Push the needle carefully forward – you may not necessarily feel the resistance going through the dura mater. If you are uncertain, check the position of the needle. Only start collecting samples with free flow of CSF. Should CSF be bloody, you have to redo the procedure – intrathecal administration should not be performed. Depending on the center, the collected volume

K. Scheinemann (✉)
Division of Hematology/Oncology, McMaster Children's Hospital,
1200 Main Street West, 555 University Avenue, Hamilton, ON, Canada L8N 3Z5
e-mail: kschein@mcmaster.ca

K. Scheinemann and A.E. Boyce (eds.), *Emergencies in Pediatric Oncology*,
DOI 10.1007/978-1-4614-1174-1_8, © Springer Science+Business Media, LLC 2012

should match the injecting volume or the desired volume for analysis. After collection of the samples (normally cytospin, glucose and protein, and maybe a culture), stabilize the needle to administer the chemotherapy. Use your thumb and index finger to hold the needle on the conus – not the needle itself as you increase risk of infection. Use your other fingers to assure the distance from the spine. Inject the chemotherapy slowly. Once injection is completed either remove LP needle and syringe in total or remove the syringe first, reinsert the stylet, and then pull the needle back. Either way, be aware that you are dealing with chemotherapeutic waste. Postprocedure patients should be put in Trendelenburg for optimal distribution of the chemotherapy.

Most children recover very quickly from the procedure.

Lumbar puncture technique and intrathecal chemotherapy administration (Figs. 8.1–8.5).

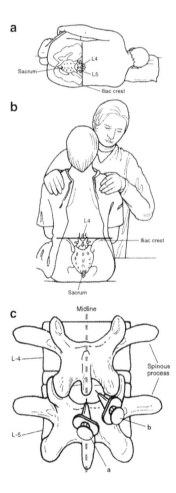

Fig. 8.1 (a) Anatomical landmarks for lumbar puncture (b) Right position of the LP needle after insertion (c)

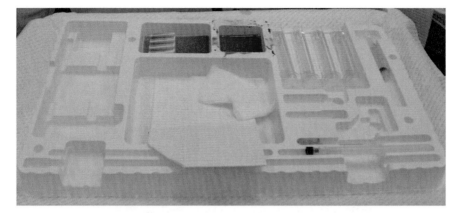

Fig. 8.2 Lumbar puncture procedure tray-at least two tubes of CSF should be collected for cytospin, glucose and total cell count

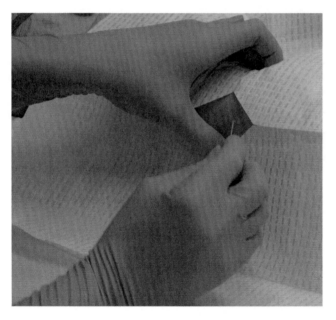

Fig. 8.3 Insertion of LP needle after verifying of landmarks, use your thumb as marker for the vertebral body

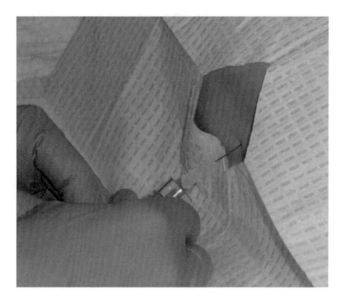

Fig. 8.4 Collection of CSF-LP needle is stable

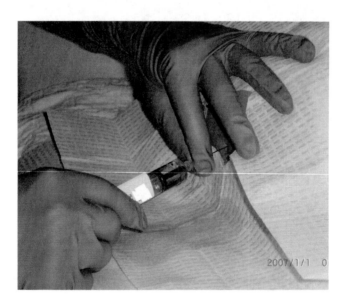

Fig. 8.5 Injection of intrathecal chemotherapy-very important to stabilize the needle against the body and only to touch the conus of the LP needle

Bone marrow aspiration and biopsy.

Bone marrow aspiration and biopsies are performed quite often for diagnostic purposes and staging. Often, other services are requesting a bone marrow investigation prior to starting systemic steroids to "rule out malignancy."

Patients/parents should have consented to this invasive procedure. Common side effects include local pain or bone pain and infection/cellulitis.

Patients are positioned in the left or right (depending on performing person's dexterity) lateral position. The area is prepped in an aseptic technique. After location of the posterior superior iliac spine, local anesthetic can be injected depending on performer's preference. Other possible location for a bone marrow aspiration is the anterior superior iliac spine. The aspiration needle then should be inserted in a 90-degree angle from the skin. Once the needle is no longer loose, aspiration of fluid can be performed. If not successful, the needle should be repositioned – correction should be in the distal direction. Sometimes the aspiration needle is too thin, and then an attempt with a biopsy needle should be done. The amount of samples should be calculated prior to the procedure. Sometimes a trephine biopsy is needed. Indications are "dry tap," assessment of cellularity, and infiltration of bone marrow through metastatic tumors or protocol requirement. The technique is the same. The needle is inserted until stuck, then the stylet should be removed and the needle further advanced at least 1 cm. To loosen the biopsy cylinder, either the needle should be turned multiple times clockwise and anti-clockwise or shaken. After loosening the cylinder, it is important to pull back in one movement – please alert the people holding the patient. Whether the biopsy is sufficient or not can be assessed immediately (Figs. 8.6–8.10). Please note that children recover very quickly from this procedure, and complaints about bone pain post procedure are rare.

Bone marrow aspiration and biopsy technique.

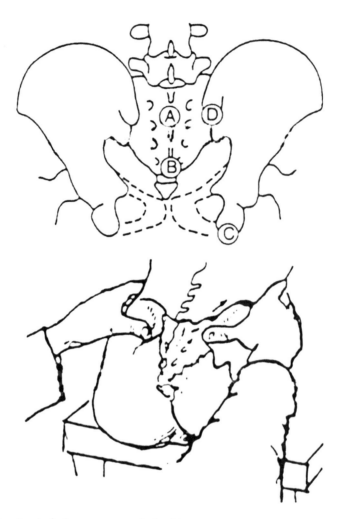

Fig. 8.6 Landmarks for bone marrow aspiration/biopsy

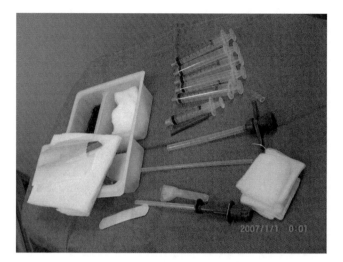

Fig. 8.7 Procedure tray: bone marrow aspiration needle (*bottom*), bone marrow biopsy needle (*top*)

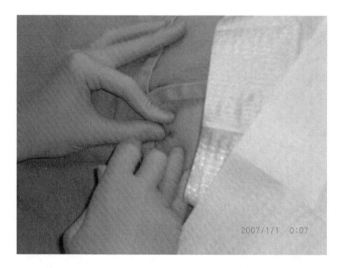

Fig. 8.8 Insertion of aspiration needle after verifying the landmarks

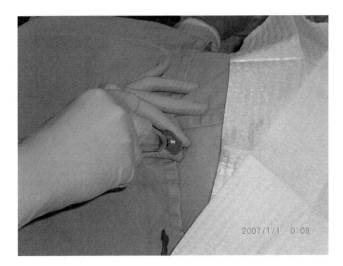

Fig. 8.9 Aspiration of bone marrow (important to fixate the needle and the syringe)

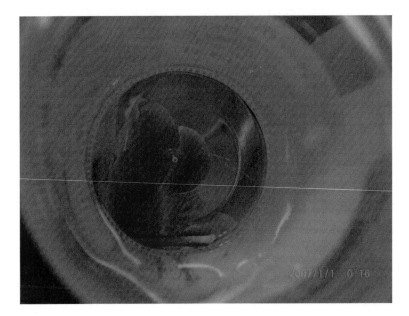

Fig. 8.10 Bone marrow biopsy

Chapter 9
Blood and Blood Product Transfusions

Stephanie Cox

Keywords ABO antibodies • Allergic reactions • Bleeding complications • CMV seronegative products • Febrile reactions • Guideline for platelet transfusion • Infusion time • Irradiation • Monitoring • Platelet transfusions • Platelets • Red blood cells • Rh immune globulin • Transfusion guidelines • Transfusion reactions

Overview

Red blood cells (RBCs) and platelets are a vital resource to support pediatric patients undergoing chemotherapy and radiation treatments. An epidemiologic study assessing blood and blood product transfusion in children found that RBCs and platelets were the two most frequently transfused products, and the rates of transfusion were highest among children with neutropenia and agranulocytosis [1]. The same study found that complications associated with blood product transfusion were rare, with a complication rate of 10.7 per 1,000 units transfused [1]. This chapter will discuss RBC and platelet transfusions in pediatric oncology patients, special product requirements, complications, and management of transfusion reactions.

Informed Consent

The administration of blood and blood products requires a discussion with the patient and caregivers to obtain informed consent. The discussion must include a description of the blood or blood product, benefits of transfusion, risks involved

S. Cox (✉)
Division of Hematology/Oncology, McMaster Children's Hospital
1280 Main Street West, Hamilton, ON, Canada L8S 4K1
e-mail: coxst@hhsc.ca

K. Scheinemann and A.E. Boyce (eds.), *Emergencies in Pediatric Oncology*,
DOI 10.1007/978-1-4614-1174-1_9, © Springer Science+Business Media, LLC 2012

with the transfusion, notably infectious risks, and possible alternatives to the transfusion. An opportunity for the patient and caregivers to ask questions must be provided. Institutional requirements for the informed consent procedure should be followed.

Red Blood Cell Transfusion (PRBC)

Red blood cells are commonly referred to as packed cells, red cells, packed red blood cells, or RBCs. RBCs consist of erythrocytes concentrated from whole-blood donations by centrifugation or collected by the apheresis method [2]. RBCs must be compatible with ABO antibodies present in the recipient serum. Each recipient and unit must be crossmatched to confirm compatibility.

Properties of each unit include [2]:

- Citrate as anticoagulants
- One or more preservatives added
- An average of 50 mL of donor plasma
- Hematocrit from 50 to 80%
- 128–240 mL of pure red cells
- 147–278 mg of iron

Indications

For children with *symptomatic* deficiency of oxygen carrying capacity or tissue hypoxia due to an inadequate circulating red cell mass [2]. As always, transfusion decisions must be made on an individual patient basis. Typical signs and symptoms of anemia requiring transfusion include pallor, malaise, irritability, and/or lassitude. Children receiving radiation therapy should be transfused more aggressively to maximize the effect of radiation by improving oxygenation of the tumor bed [3].

General transfusion guidelines include [4]:

- Hemoglobin 70–100 g/L – transfuse if with signs and symptoms of impaired oxygen delivery.
- Hemoglobin <70 g/L – appropriate to transfuse.
- Hemoglobin <60 g/L – transfusion highly recommended.

Dosing

- 10–15 mL/kg is generally given.

Infusion Time

A transfusion rate of approximately 2.5 mL/kg/h usually avoids circulatory overload. The average transfusion time will range from 2 to 4 h. Patients with cardiovascular instability may require a slower transfusion rate greater than 4 h.

Monitoring

The patient requires close monitoring throughout the transfusion.
   Vital signs should be monitored:

- At the start of the transfusion
- 15 min into the transfusion
- Regular intervals per hospital policy
- The completion of transfusion
- As necessary, if any signs or symptoms of transfusion reaction

Anticipated Response

The hemoglobin concentration will usually rise by 2–3 gm/dL or the hematocrit by 6–9% if the concentration of red cells is approximately 65% [5].

Platelet Transfusion

Platelet transfusions are commonly referred to as platelets pooled, random donor platelets (RDP), platelets pheresis, and single-donor platelets (SDP). When possible, RDPs and SDPs should be ABO identical to the recipient, but it is not necessary when unavailable. As well, Rh-negative recipients should receive Rh-negative platelets. However, when this is not available, consider administering Rh-immune globulin.
   Properties of each unit of RDPs include [2]:

- $\geq 5.5 \times 10^{10}$ platelets (average 8.0×10^{10}) per bag.
- Approximately 50 mL of plasma.
- Anticoagulant, the same as used for whole-blood collection.
- 4–10 units are pooled prior to transfusion to prepare an adult dose.

   Properties of each unit of SDPs include [2]:

- $\geq 3.0 \times 10^{11}$ platelets (average 3.5–4.0×10^{11}) per bag.
- Approximately 250 mL of plasma.
- SDPs are ready for transfusion.

Indications

Platelet transfusions are indicated to treat bleeding due to decreased circulating platelets or functionally abnormal platelets. As well, platelets are used prophylactically as specified thresholds to prevent bleeding complications. The 2010 guideline for platelet transfusion thresholds for pediatric oncology patients published by the C17 Standards and Guidelines Committee include [6]:

Please check institutional guidelines first – these are only recommendations.

- Clinically stable patients receiving chemotherapy for leukemia, post–stem cell transplantation, or patients with solid tumors → 10×10^9 per L
- Stable patients requiring lumbar puncture → 20×10^9 per L (more common 50×10^9 per L)
- Newly diagnosed patients with leukemia for diagnostic LP to minimize risk of traumatic LP → 50×10^9 per L
- Patients with leukemia/lymphoma with signs of bleeding, high fever, hyperleukocytosis, rapid fall in platelet count, acute promyelocytic leukemia, coagulation abnormality, critically ill patients, and impaired platelet function → 40×10^9 per L
- Stable patients requiring major invasive procedure → $40–50 \times 10^9$ per L
- Child has a CNS tumor with:

  - VP shunt or Ommaya reservoir → 30×10^9 per L
  - Past history of ICH → 50×10^9 per L
  - Infant receiving intensive chemotherapy → 30×10^9 per L
  - Undergoing neurosurgical procedure → 100×10^9 per L
  - Gross total resection or residual tumor and receiving chemotherapy and/or radiation → 30×10^9 per L
  - Receiving antiangiogenesis agent → 50×10^9 per L
  - Undergo LP with past history of CNS tumor → 50×10^9 per L

Dosing

Based on institutional blood bank guidelines, but generally includes:

- 5–10 mL/kg up to maximum 300 mL (adult dose)
- 1 unit RDP per 10 kg up to 5 units (adult dose)
- 1 unit of SDP is equivalent to 5 units RDP

Infusion Time

Based on institutional standards but generally includes:

- 20–60-min infusion time

Monitoring

The patient requires close monitoring throughout the transfusion.
    Vital signs should be monitored:

- At the start of the transfusion
- 15 min into the transfusion
- At the completion of transfusion
- As necessary, if any signs or symptoms of transfusion reaction

Anticipated Response

A transfusion of 5–10 mL/kg of RDP should produce an increase in platelet count of 50–100,000 per mm^3. For unit-based dosing, an expected rise of 7,000–10,000 per mm^3 for each unit of RDP given or 30,000–60,000 per mm^3 for each unit of SDP [2]. However, the response from a platelet transfusion can be adversely affected by high-grade fever, sepsis, splenomegaly, severe bleeding, consumptive coagulopathy, HLA alloimmunization, and treatment with certain drugs notably amphotericin B [2]. A post-platelet count drawn from 10 min to 3 h posttransfusion can be helpful in detecting adequate response or alloimmunization refractory patients.

Special Product Requirements

RBC and platelet transfusions are capable of transmitting cytomegalovirus (CMV), mediating transfusion-associated graft versus host disease (TA-GvHD) and causing febrile, nonhemolytic reactions. For pediatric oncology patients who are at risk for these complications due to repeated exposure to transfusions, many institutions will provide special blood products including gamma-irradiated and CMV-seronegative products.

Irradiation

Irradiation of the blood component renders T lymphocytes incapable of proliferation and is presently the only approved means to prevent TA-GvHD [2]. Patients at risk who should receive irradiated products include [4]:

- Patients with hematologic malignancies, including lymphoma and leukemia
- Patients undergoing bone marrow or stem cell transplantation
- Patients with solid tumors undergoing aggressive or myeloablative chemotherapy

CMV-seronegative products

Of the blood donors, 40–70% may be CMV positive, and leukoreduction removes most but not all CMV from blood components [2, 4]. CMV transmission can be harmful to patients who are significantly immunocompromised including allogeneic bone marrow transplant recipients. The risk of transmission can be reduced by providing CMV-seronegative products to these high-risk patients.

Noninfectious Complications

Acute <24h Transfusion Reactions (Tables 9.1 and 9.2)
Delayed >24 h Transfusion Reactions (Tables 9.3 and 9.4)

Table 9.1 Immunologic [2, 4]

Complication	Risk of event	Etiology
Hemolytic	1 in 40,000	Destruction of transfused red cells due to ABO incompatibility
Febrile nonhemolytic reaction	1 in 10 per 5 RDP units 1 in 300 per unit RBC	Temperature $\uparrow \geq 1\,°C$ occurring during or shortly after transfusion due to antibody to donor leukocytes or action of cytokines
Allergic reaction	1 in 100 (urticaria)	Urticarial but may also include wheezing or angioedema reactions due to antibodies to donor plasma proteins
Anaphylactic reaction	1 in 40,000 per unit of component	Autonomic dysregulation, severe dyspnea, pulmonary and/or laryngeal edema, and bronchospasm due to antibodies to donor plasma proteins
Transfusion-related acute lung injury	1 in 5,000	$\uparrow$ permeability of the pulmonary microcirculation causes massive leakage of fluids and protein into alveolar spaces usually within 6 h of transfusion

Table 9.2 Nonimmunologic [2, 4]

Complication	Risk of event	Etiology
Circulatory overload	1 in 700 per transfusion episode	Volume overload
Transfusion-associated sepsis	1 in 10,000 symptomatic bacterial sepsis per pool of 5 RDP 1 in 100,000 symptomatic bacterial sepsis per unit RBC	Onset of high fever with temp $\uparrow$ ≥ 2 C, severe chills, hypotension, or circulatory collapse during or immediately after transfusion suggest bacterial contamination or endotoxin reaction

Table 9.3 Immunologic [2, 4]

Complication	Risk of event	Etiology
Alloimmunization	1 in 100	Development of antigens to RBCs or platelets may occur unpredictably after transfusion
Hemolytic	1 in 7,000	Often patients are asymptomatic but develop anamnestic immune response to RBC antigens
TA-GvHD	Rare	Extremely dangerous condition occurs when viable T lymphocytes in the transfused component engraft in the recipient and react against tissue antigens in the recipient
Posttransfusion purpura	Rare	Development of sudden and self-limiting thrombocytopenia 7 to 10 days posttransfusion

Table 9.4 Infectious complications [2, 4]

Infectious complication	Risk of event per unit of treatment
Death from bacterial sepsis per pool 5 RDP platelets	1 in 40,000
Transmission of hepatitis B	1 in 82,000
Death from bacterial sepsis per unit of RBC	1 in 100,000
Transmission of West Nile virus	<1 in 1,000,000
Transmission of HTLV	1 in 3,000,000
Transmission of hepatitis C	1 in 3,100,000
Transmission of HIV	1 in 4,700,000

Management of Transfusion Reactions

All transfusion reactions should be reported to your hospital's transfusion service and institutional policies followed. Patients and caregivers should be instructed to notify their nurse if they experience hives or itching, feeling feverish or chills, difficulty breathing, back pain or pain at the infusion site, or any feeling different from usual.

General guidelines for suspected transfusion reactions [4]:

1. STOP the transfusion
2. Maintain IV access
3. Check vital signs
4. Recheck patient ID band and product label
5. Notify physician
6. Notify transfusion laboratory

1. Febrile reactions – are defined as a temperature increase of $\geq 1°C$ and temperature $>38°C$ during transfusion or within 4 h of completion of transfusion.

   (a) If patient symptoms include temperature $\geq 39°C$, hypotension, tachycardia, rigors/chills, anxiety, dyspnea, back/chest pain, or nausea and vomiting:

   - Possible hemolytic reaction or bacterial contamination – discontinue transfusion, collect samples from product, and draw blood cultures.

(b) If patient does not have above symptoms:

- Likely febrile nonhemolytic reaction – administer acetaminophen and continue transfusion cautiously.

2. Allergic reactions – are defined as presence of urticaria, facial edema, airway edema, lower respiratory tract symptoms, hypotension, or shock.

(a) If patient symptoms include hypotension, dyspnea/cough, tachycardia, generalized flushing or anxiety, nausea and vomiting, or widespread rash $\geq 2/3$ of body surface area:

- Possible severe allergic or anaphylactic reaction – treat with diphenhydramine, corticosteroids, and epinephrine as required and do NOT restart transfusion.

(b) If patient does not have above symptoms:

- Likely minor allergic reaction – administer diphenhydramine and continue transfusion cautiously.

Pretreatment for Recurrent Reactions

- For patients with recurrent febrile, nonhemolytic reactions:
  - Premedicate with acetaminophen.
- For patients with recurrent urticarial reactions:
  - Premedicate with diphenhydramine and/or corticosteroids, and request plasma depletion, washed RBCs, or platelets.

References

1. Slonim, A. Blood transfusions in children: a multi-institutional analysis of practices and complications. Transfusion. 2008., 48(1): 73–80.
2. American National Red Cross. Practice guidelines for blood transfusion: A compilation from recent peer-reviewed literature. (2nd ed). 2007, http://www.aabb.org.
3. Teruya, J. Indications for red blood cell transfusion in infants and children. In: UpToDate, Mahoney, D. (Ed), UpToDate, Waltham, MA, 2011.
4. Callum, J. and Pinkerton, P. Bloody easy 2: Blood transfusions, blood alternatives and transfusion reactions. A guide to transfusion medicine (2nd ed). 2005. Sunnybrook & Women's College Health Sciences Centre.
5. Teruya, J. Administration and complications of red cell transfusion in infants and children. In: UpToDate, Mahoney, D. (Ed), UpToDate, Waltham, MA, 2011.
6. Barnard, D., Portwine, C. and Members of the C17 Standards and Guidelines Group. Guideline for platelet transfusion thresholds for pediatric oncology patients. C17 Council; Children's Cancer & Blood Disorders. Edmonton; 2010.

Chapter 10
Thromboembolism in Children with Cancer

Uma Athale and Anthony Chan

Keywords Anticoagulation therapy • Antithrombin • Asparaginase • Cerebral sinovenous thrombosis • Pulmonary embolism • Right atrial thrombosis • Thromboembolism • Thromboprophylaxis

Introduction

Thromboembolism (TE) is an uncommon problem in children. However, children with cancer have an increased risk of developing TE. A recent study in children with cancers showed overall 8% prevalence of TE compared to 0.7–1.4 events per 100,000 children in the general pediatric population [1–3]. Thrombosis associated with cancer is a multifactorial condition resulting from interaction of cancer, its therapy, and inherent host factors. Figure 10.1 depicts the proposed interaction of various factors responsible for development of cancer-related thrombosis.

Anatomical Site of Thrombosis

The sites of TE vary to some extent according to the type of cancer. For example, cerebral sinovenous thrombosis (CSVT) is common in children with ALL, whereas a large pelvic sarcoma may induce lower limb deep venous thrombosis (DVT) [4]. Upper venous system DVTs are commonly reported in association with central venous line (CVL) [5]. Chapters 12 and 13 will discuss CVL-related thrombosis

U. Athale (✉) • A. Chan
Division of Hematology/Oncology, McMaster Children's Hospital,
Hamilton, ON, Canada L8S 4K1
e-mail: athaleu@mcmaster.ca

K. Scheinemann and A.E. Boyce (eds.), *Emergencies in Pediatric Oncology*,
DOI 10.1007/978-1-4614-1174-1_10, © Springer Science+Business Media, LLC 2012

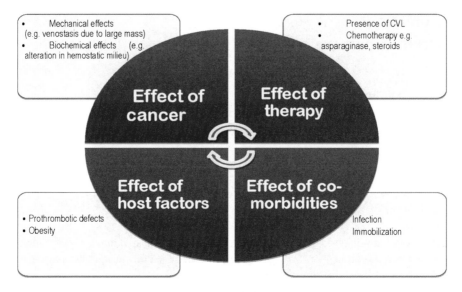

Fig. 10.1 Thrombosis in relation to cancer is a multifactorial condition resulting from interaction of various factors. Cancer, the anticancer therapy, complications related to cancer and its therapy as well as inherent patient factors may contribute to the development of prothrombotic state

Table 10.1 Proposed risk factor predisposing children with cancer to the development of thromboembolism

Factor	Risk
Type of cancer	Children with ALL, lymphoma, and sarcoma are shown to be at increased risk of symptomatic TE, whereas children with brain tumor have a very low risk of TE [1]
Age of the patient	Older children compared to younger children have increased risk of TE [1, 4, 9, 14, 18]
Presence of central venous line	Most important risk factor [2, 3]
Chemotherapy	Drugs like asparaginase and steroids are shown to be prothrombotic [4, 9, 14]
Mediastinal mass	Presence of mediastinal mass is associated with increased risk of TE [1]
Associated infection	Presence of infection is associated with increased risk of TE, especially CVL related
Inherited prothrombotic disorder	Available information is inconclusive [4, 9, 14]

ALL acute lymphoblastic leukemia; *TE* thromboembolism; *CVL* central venous line

and CSVT, respectively. In this section, we will review the available information regarding the epidemiology of TE in children with cancer, diagnosis of TE, and principles of anticoagulation management in children receiving cancer chemotherapy.

Table 10.1 outlines the proposed risk factors predisposing children with cancer to the development of TE.

Deep Venous Thrombosis

Although the presence of a CVL is identified as the most important predisposing factor for thrombosis in children, over 40% of children with cancer and symptomatic TE have thrombosis at sites distant from their CVL [6, 7]. About 10% of patients will have involvement of multiple sites at the time of the diagnosis of TE.

Right Atrial Thrombosis

Right atrial thrombosis (RAT), although uncommon, is a potentially lethal site of thrombosis. In majority of patients, RAT is related to the indwelling CVL. Presence of catheter tip in the right atrium is identified to be a major risk factor for the development of RAT [4, 8].

Overall, 2% of patients with ALL and symptomatic TE were reported to have developed RAT [6, 9]. However, studies evaluating patients for asymptomatic TE report higher (14%) prevalence of RAT [5, 6]. Korones et al. reported 8.8% prevalence of RAT in children with cancer and indwelling catheters; children with ALL were at significantly higher risk for developing RAT [10]. In a review of literature describing 122 children with RAT, 19% had cancer [11]. About 44% of patients with RAT were symptomatic; respiratory distress was the commonest symptom. Other clinical presentations include rhythm disturbances (bradycardia or tachyarrythmia), new murmur, cyanosis, hemoptysis, heart failure, or cardiac arrest (Table 10.2) [11]. For asymptomatic patients, the thrombus is usually detected on routine testing, like an echocardiogram (ECHO).

About one third of children with RAT tend to be at high risk for development of pulmonary embolism (PE) and tend to have high-risk features which include large (>2 cm in diameter) clots, pedunculated or snake-shaped clots, and mobile clots [11]. Complications of RAT include pulmonary embolism (PE) and death.

Management of RAT is usually a multidisciplinary approach involving hematologists, cardiologists, cardiothoracic surgeons, and/or interventional radiologists. Severity of associated symptoms and cardiac morbidity usually dictate the management of RAT [4, 8]. The various treatment modalities include surgical thrombectomy, thrombolysis with or without systemic anticoagulation, or systemic anticoagulation alone. Surgical thrombectomy or thrombolysis with or without systemic anticoagulation is usually indicated for high-risk clots, whereas systemic anticoagulation, CVL removal, or observation alone are modalities suitable for low-risk clots. For either therapeutic choices, close monitoring with frequent ECHO is essential. More aggressive surgical approach may result in delay in chemotherapy, and thrombolysis may lead to pulmonary embolism.

Pulmonary Embolism

In general, pulmonary embolism is rare in children. Two recent childhood thrombosis registries reported annual incidence of PE ranging from 0.14 to 0.9 cases per 100,000 children [2, 3]. A recent study from the Hospital for Sick Children, Toronto, reported a much higher prevalence of PE of 4.6/100,000 children [11]. In this study, cancer (occurring with a frequency of ~18%) was the second most important underlying disease in children with PE. The reported frequency of PE in children with cancer varies from 0.5% to 2.9% [1, 11, 12]. However, in a cohort of 55 children with cancer and symptomatic thrombosis, PE was present in 5% of patients [1].

Risk Factors Predisposing to the Development of PE

This information is mainly based on studies in general pediatric population [11, 13]. Idiopathic PE is rare in childhood. Almost all patients have an underlying risk factor:

1. Presence of CVL: One study identified PE in 16% of patients with CVL. Despite higher prevalence of CVL-associated upper extremity thrombosis in children with ALL, PE is reported only in ~2% of children with ALL and symptomatic TE [4, 6]
2. Concurrent DVT: About 70% of children with PE are reported to have clots elsewhere in the body
3. Cardiac disease: The most common underlying condition in children with PE
4. Recent surgery
5. Immobilization
6. Prothrombotic defects: Identified in ~30% of children with PE

Complications and Outcome of PE

PE is a serious condition with ~9% fatality rate. Systemic anticoagulation is effective in complete or partial resolution of PE in ~80% of children. However, bleeding is a common complication reported in ~20% of children. Recurrence of PE is also common especially with recurrence of predisposing risk factors. Pulmonary hypertension is a significant problem in survivors of PE.

Evaluation of a Child with Suspected Thromboembolism

Clinical presentation depends on the age of the patients, site of thrombosis, extent of occlusion, and acuteness of occlusion. Although the clinical symptoms of thrombosis in children with cancer are usually similar to those seen in patients without malignancy, the clinical presentation of thrombosis may be complicated by other cancer-associated comorbidities and may delay the diagnosis of TE. For example, headache secondary to CSVT in a child receiving antileukemic therapy may be attributed to intrathecal chemotherapy or hypertension secondary to steroid therapy. This may delay the diagnosis of CSVT. Hence, a high index of suspicion is essential.

Diagnosis of TE should be objectively confirmed by at least one (or more) diagnostic method. In the presence of TE at one site, it is recommended that other sites be evaluated (especially if anatomically related, e.g., jugular vessels in the presence of cerebral sinovenous thrombosis) for associated asymptomatic TE at other site. Table 10.2 outlines common symptoms associated with various types of TE and recommended investigations to confirm thrombosis.

Management of Thrombosis in Children with Cancer

So far, there are no evidence-based guidelines for prevention and management of TE in children with cancer. Most of the recommendations are based on studies conducted either in the general pediatric population or in adults with cancer [4, 14]. We refer the reader to a more extensive review on this subject [15].

Anticoagulation Therapy in Children with Cancer

Thrombocytopenia and coagulopathy which are commonly present in children receiving chemotherapy can increase the risk of bleeding associated with anticoagulation therapy. Further, invasive procedures (e.g., lumbar puncture with/without chemotherapy, bone marrow aspiration and biopsy, tissue biopsy, second-look surgery, or neurosurgery) are an inherent part of cancer therapy. Conservative anticothrombotic management has the danger of progression of thrombosis or residual thrombosis, whereas aggressive therapy may lead to bleeding. These factors pose special challenges in the management of a child with cancer requiring anticoagulation therapy.

Here, we will discuss the challenges posed by the use of anticoagulation therapy in children receiving chemotherapy and the special considerations required for treating children with cancer.

Choice of Anticoagulant Agent

The details of antithrombotic agents are beyond the scope of this chapter. We refer the reader to more extensive reference on this topic [15]. Table 10.3 refers to the advantages and disadvantages of different anticoagulation agents with special reference

Table 10.2 Evaluation and diagnosis for patients with suspected thrombosis

	Site	Likely clinical signs and symptoms	Diagnostic method/s
CNS	Arterial ischemic stroke ± hemorrhage	Unexplained headaches, vomiting, visual problems or neurological deficits, seizure, drowsiness or any change in mental status, signs of raised intracranial pressure	MRI/MRA Angiogram
	Sinovenous thrombosis (SVT)		MRI/MRV CT venogram
PE	Pulmonary vasculature	Respiratory problems (shortness of breath, tachypnea, dyspnea), bradycardia, tachyarrythmia, cardiac failure, hypoxia, chest pain, syncope, "unexplained pneumonia"	V/Q scan Spiral CT Pulmonary angiogram
DVT	Upper venous system	Swelling, pain, tenderness, erythema, dilated vessels	Bilateral venogram is a "gold standard" for diagnosis of subclavian/brachial vessels TE Doppler USG necessary for jugular vein TE[a] MRV Recommend ECHO to evaluate RAT
	Lower venous system		Doppler USG to evaluate all sites[a] Venogram is still the gold standard
Cardiac	Right atrial	CVL occlusion, sepsis, congestive heart failure	ECHO
CVL related DVT	At or near CVL	Swelling, pain, tenderness, erythema, dilated vessels, CVL occlusion requiring revision or renewal, headache, swelling of face Red flags: recurrent CVL-related infections A significant CVL-related DVT of the vessel harboring CVL may be asymptomatic. Hence, high index of suspicion is required	ECHO, linogram, venogram and/or Doppler USG depending upon the site of thrombosis[a]

[a] Detection of echogenic material within the lumen of a vein on a gray scale and presence of partial or complete absence of flow by pulse wave or color Doppler ultrasonography

TE thromboembolism; *CNS* central nervous system; *MRI* magnetic resonance imaging; *MRV* magnetic resonance venogram; *MRA* magnetic resonance arteriogram; *PE* pulmonary embolism; *V/Q scan* ventilation/perfusion scan; *CT* computerized tomography; *DVT* deep venous thrombosis; *USG* ultrasonogram; *CVL* central venous line; *RAT* right atrial thrombosis; *ECHO* echocardiography

Adapted from Wiernikowski J, Athale UH. Thromboembolic complications in children with cancer. Thrombosis research 2006;118:137-152

Table 10.3 Summary of various anticoagulant agents available for treatment of children with cancer

Anticoagulant	Monitoring	Advantages	Disadvantages/complications	Special considerations for children with cancer
Unfractionated heparin (UFH)	aPTT Difficult monitoring	Easy reversal	Bleeding Osteoporosis	Bleeding may be exaggerated due to thrombocytopenia and coagulopathy Osteoporosis may be exaggerated in children treated with glucocorticoids (e.g., ALL, NHL)
Low-molecular-weight heparin (LMWH)	Anti-Xa levels Easy monitoring	Efficacy comparable to UFH and safe Cost effective	Subcutaneous administration Bleeding complication (0–5.6%)	Target anti-Xa levels in children are unknown Difficult to reverse anticoagulation in emergency situation
Oral anticoagulants	INR Difficult monitoring	Oral administration Low cost	Dose requirements strongly influenced by age Efficacy affected by diet[a] No stability data on solution or suspension, making dosing in young children and in children unable to swallow tablets difficult	Dietary alterations (due to mucositis, TPN) and antibacterial therapy (PCP prophylaxis or treatment for fever and neutropenia) lead to unpredictable exogenous and endogenous Vitamin K levels Warfarin metabolism by cytochrome P450 system leading to numerous drug interactions with anticancer agents (e.g., corticosteroids)

[a] Babies may have resistance to warfarin if formula fed (vitamin K enriched), whereas breastfed infants may be oversensitive due to poor vitamin K content in breast milk

UFH unfractionated heparin; *aPTT* activated partial thromboplastin time; *ALL* acute lymphoblastic leukemia; *NHL* non-Hodgkin's lymphoma; *LMWH* low-molecular-weight heparin; *INR* international normalization ratio; *TPN* total parenteral nutrition; *PCP Pneumocystis carinii* pneumonia
Adapted from Athale UH, Chan AKC. Thromboembolic complications in pediatric hematologic malignancies. Semin Thromb Hemost 2007, 33:416-26

to children with cancer [4, 14, 15]. Low-molecular-weight heparin (LMWH) is safe, as effective as unfractionated heparin (UFH), has minimal drug interactions, and is easy to manage around elective invasive procedures. Hence, LMWH is the preferred anticoagulant in children with cancer. The dosing is adjusted to achieve an anti-Xa activity between 0.5 and 1.0 U/dL.

Management of Anticoagulation Therapy Around Invasive Procedures

Due to the risk of bleeding and spinal hematomas, it is recommended to withhold at least two doses of LMWH and to determine anti-Xa levels prior to surgical procedure, if possible, prior to lumbar puncture or epidural procedures [15]. In some facilities, LMWH is held for 24 h prior to LP or surgical procedures. However, it may not be routine to check anti-Xa level prior to the procedure. LMWH is resumed soon after the procedure if the procedure is uncomplicated. Following a more invasive procedure (like surgery), anticoagulation can be started after consultation with surgical colleagues and only when the risk of bleeding is deemed to be minimal or nonexistent.

Management of Anticoagulation Therapy in the Presence of Thrombocytopenia

There are no evidence-based guidelines for dose adjustment of anticoagulation therapy in relation to platelet counts.

In absence of any other coagulopathy, we use following guidelines:

- Full-dose LMWH therapy for patients with platelet count $>30 \times 10^9$ per L.
- 50% of dose at a platelet count between 20 and 30×10^9 per L.
- Withhold LMWH for platelet count $<20 \times 10^9$ per L.

In early stages of thrombosis or thrombosis in organ or life-threatening sites (e.g., CSVT, PE), it is important to maximize the anticoagulation therapy. In these circumstances, platelet transfusions are given prior to anticoagulation to maximize the anticoagulation in patients with thrombocytopenia. If at all possible, it is preferred to have uninterrupted anticoagulation during the first month of antithrombotic therapy.

A close monitoring of platelet count and careful watching for signs of bleeding are necessary. Depending on anticipated drop in platelet count, we check platelet counts either daily or twice/three times a week.

Please note: These practice guidelines are based on personal experience.

Management of Asparaginase Therapy in a Child with TE

In conditions treated with asparaginase (e.g., acute lymphoblastic leukemia, lymphoma), the development of thrombosis is closely associated with asparaginase therapy. Asparaginase is shown to reduce synthesis of natural anticoagulants especially antithrombin (AT) resulting in an acquired prothrombotic state. Other drugs like steroids also induce a prothrombotic state and increase the risk of thrombosis in patients receiving combination chemotherapy. Since asparaginase seems to be the main culprit, development of TE warrants temporary withholding of asparaginase therapy. However, asparaginase is an important component of antileukemic therapy, and interruption of asparaginase therapy is shown to affect outcome from ALL [16]. Hence, it is important to make every effort to resume asparaginase once anticoagulation therapy is established. The currently safe and effective anticoagulation therapy makes it possible to continue asparaginase therapy with concomitant anticoagulation, and there is no need for permanent discontinuation of asparaginase.

In a child diagnosed with symptomatic or clinically significant thrombosis, we recommend initiating anticoagulation therapy, if no bleeding risk, and withholding further asparaginase therapy until the clinical condition stabilizes and hematological parameters normalize. Once TE is under control and the anti-Xa levels are in the desirable range, we reinstate asparaginase along with continuation of anticoagulant therapy. We continue anticoagulation therapy for at least 3 months or until 3–4 weeks after completion of asparaginase therapy, whichever is longer.

Role of Antithrombin Replacement in Patients on Asparaginase Therapy

Acquired antithrombin (AT) deficiency is thought to be the main pathogenic mechanism for asparaginase-induced prothrombotic state. Hence, it is intuitive to consider AT replacement along with asparaginase therapy. However, the clinical benefit of routine AT supplementation in prevention of TE is yet to be proven, and so far, there are no data to support routine use of FFP or AT supplementation in children receiving asparaginase [4, 5, 14]. Despite lack of evidence, several institutions continue to supplement FFP and/or AT for prevention of thrombosis while receiving asparaginase. This practice may lead to unnecessary exposure to blood products.

Reduction in AT levels may influence the efficacy of heparin based anticoagulation therapy. For patients on LMWH-based anticoagulation, AT replacement is not necessary as long as targeted anti-Xa level is achieved.

Primary Thromboprophylaxis for CVL-related TE

Results of several randomized controlled trials (RCTs) do not recommend primary thromboprophylaxis for adults with malignancy for prevention of CVL-related TE [17]. Similarly, studies in children do not support the use of primary thromboprophylaxis of CVL- related TE [4, 14, 15].

Secondary Thromboprophylaxis Following Development of TE

A retrospective study and a recent population-based study showed that children with cancer are at increased risk of recurrence of TE [1, 18]. Hence, we offer secondary prophylaxis in children with cancer especially if there is reexposure to the identified risk factor (e.g., asparaginase therapy or relapse/recurrence of cancer).

References

1. Athale UH, Siciliano S, Thabane L, Pai N, Cox S, Lathia A, Khan AA, Armstrong A, Chan AKC. Epidemiology and clinical risk factors predisposing to thromboembolism in children with cancer. Pediatric Blood and Cancer, 2008; 51:792–7
2. Monagle P, Adams M, Mahoney M, et al. Outcome of pediatric thromboembolic disease: A report from the Canadian Childhood Thrombophilia Registry. Pediatric Research 2000; 47:763–6
3. van Ommen CH, Heijboer H, Baller HR, Hirasing RA, Heijmanom HSA, Peter M. Venous thromboembolism in childhood: A prospective two-year registry in The Netherlands. J Pediatr 2001; 139:676–81
4. Athale UH, Wiernikowski J. Thromboembolic complications in children with cancer. Thrombosis Research, 2006; 118:137–152
5. Mitchell LG, Andrew M, Hanna K, Abshire T, Halton J, Anderson R, Cherrick I, Desai S, Mahoney D, McCuster P, Wu J, Dahl G, Chait P, de Veber G, Lee KJ, Mikulis D, Ginsberg J, Way C. A prospective cohort study determining the prevalence of thrombotic events in children with acute lymphoblastic leukemia and a central venous line who are treated with L-asparaginase: results of the Prophylactic Antithrombin Replacement in Kids with Acute Lymphoblastic Leukemia Treated with Asparaginase (PARKAA) Study. Cancer. 2003; 97:508–516.
6. Athale UH, Chan AKC. Thrombosis in children with acute lymphoblastic leukemia Part I: Epidemiology of thrombosis in children with acute lymphoblastic leukemia. Thrombosis Research 2003; 111:125–131
7. Wermes C, Prondzinski M vD, Lichtinghagen R, Barthels M, Welte K, Sykora KW. Clinical relevance of genetic risk factors for thrombosis in pediatric oncology patients with central venous catheters. Eur J Pediatr 1999; 158 (Suppl3): S143–S146
8. Yang JYK, Williams S, Brandao LR, Chan AKC. Neonatal and childhood right atrial thrombosis: recognition and risk-stratified treatment approach Blood Coagulation and Fibirinolysis 2010; 21:301–307
9. Caruso V, Lacoviello L, Di Castelnuovo A, Storti S, Mariani G, de Gaetano G. Thrombotic complications in childhood acute lymphoblastic leukaemia: a meta-analysis of 17 prospective studies comprising 1752 pediatric patients. Blood 2006; 108:2216–2222
10. Korones DN, Buzzard CJ, Asselin B, Harris JP. Right atrial thrombi in children with cancer and indwelling catheters. J Pediatr 1996; 128:841–6
11. Biss TT, Brandao LR, Kahr WH, Chan AKC, Williams S. Clinical features and outcome of pulmonary embolism in children. British Journal of Hematology 2008; 142:808–818
12. Duero C, Facing P, Ravalli A, Arioso M, March PF, Riva A, Marino G, Baptize A, Massera G. Pulmonary embolism in childhood leukemia: 8 years' experience in pediatric hematology center. Journal of Clinical oncology 1995; 13:2805–2812
13. Van Ommen CH, Peters M. Acute pulmonary embolism in childhood. Thrombosis research 118: 13–25

14. Athale UH, Chan AKC. Thromboembolic complications in pediatric hematologic malignancies. Seminars in Thrombosis and Hemostasis 2007; 33(4): 416–426

15. Monagle P, Chalmers E, Chan AKC et al. Antithrombotic therapy in neonates and children: American College of Chest Physicians evidence-based clinical practice guidelines (8th edition) Chest 2008; 133:887–968

16. Silverman LB, Geber RD, Dalton VK, Asselin BL, Barr RD, Cavell LA, Hurwitz CA, Maghreb A, Samson Y, Schering MA, Akin S, DeClerck L, Cohen HJ, Sallan SE. Improved outcome of children with acute lymphoblastic leukemia: results of Dana-Farber consortium protocol 91-01. Blood, 2001; 97:1211–7

17. Agnelli G, Verso M. Is antithrombotic prophylaxis required in cancer patients with central venous catheters? No. J Thromb Haemost. 2006; 4:14–15

18. Raffini L, Huang Y-S, Witmer C, Feudtner C. A significant increase in venous thromboembolism in U.S. Children's Hospitals from 2001-2007. J Thromb Haemost 2009;7(2)

Chapter 11
Cerebral Sinovenous Thrombosis in Children with Cancer

Uma Athale and Anthony Chan

Keywords Cerebral sinovenous thrombosis • Cerebrovascular accidents • Duration of anticoagulation • Hypercoagulable state • ICP • Intracranial pressure • Prothrombotic disorder • Recurrent CSVT • Thrombolytic therapy • Venous infarction

Introduction

Compared to general pediatric population, children with cancer are at increased risk of cerebral sinovenous thrombosis (CSVT). CSVT is associated with high morbidity and mortality. Hence, early detection and prompt therapy is essential.

A recent study has shown an increased risk of thromboembolic events including cerebral sinus venous thrombosis in children with cancer [1]. This probably is related to aggressive and more invasive therapies, increased awareness, and improved imaging techniques. In 2001, Canadian Pediatric Stroke Registry noted an incidence of CSVT to be 0.7 cases per 100,000 children per year [2]. Raiser et al. recently reported CSVT in 0.3% of patients seen in neurologic consultation [3]. Wermes et al. reported ~6% incidence of CSVT in children with acute lymphoblastic leukemia (ALL) treated on Berlin–Frankfurt–Munster (BFM) ALL 90/95 protocol [4]. The predisposition to the development of CSVT varies with the type of cancer and the chemotherapy protocol used as well as underlying factors.

U. Athale (✉) • A. Chan
Division of Hematology/Oncology, McMaster Children's Hospital,
Hamilton, ON, Canada L8S 4K1
e-mail: athaleu@mcmaster.ca

K. Scheinemann and A.E. Boyce (eds.), *Emergencies in Pediatric Oncology*,
DOI 10.1007/978-1-4614-1174-1_11, © Springer Science+Business Media, LLC 2012

CSVT in Children with Cancer

Cerebrovascular accidents including thromboembolism are one of the common causes of acute neurologic deterioration in children with cancer [5]. About half of the children with ALL and symptomatic thrombosis have central nervous system (CNS) thrombosis, and over half of these CNS thromboses occur in the cerebral sinovenous area [6–8]. This may be related to the use of asparaginase in most ALL therapy protocols.

However, CSVT has also been reported in children with cancers other than ALL. CSVT has been reported in patients with non-Hodgkin's lymphoma (NHL) with or without asparaginase therapy [9, 10]. It is estimated that ~1–3% of patients with NHL may develop CSVT. Other childhood tumors such as neuroblastoma have also been reported in association with CSVT [9].

Anatomy of Cerebral Sinovenous System and Pathogenesis of CSVT

Figure 11.1 depicts the anatomy of the cerebral sinovenous system. In CSVT, thrombosis occurs both in veins of brain and venous sinuses. The thrombosis of the brain veins lead to venous infarction leading to insufficient blood supply and venous congestion. This in turn results in cerebral edema (both vasogenic and cyto-toxic). Vasogenic edema results mostly from venous congestion and cytotoxic edema probably due to ischemia as a result of reduced blood flow. The venous congestion may lead to small petechial hemorrhages which may merge into large hematomas.

The thrombosis of venous sinuses leads to reduced absorption of cerebrospinal fluid (CSF) and an increase in intracranial pressure (ICP). Figure 11.2 outlines the CSF flow and absorption into the venous system via arachnoid granulation. Thus, CSVT leads to CSF blockage and raised ICP, usually without ventricular dilatation. Based on the severity and acuity of obstruction, the raised ICP could be asymptom-atic or even fatal.

CSVT may occur in superficial or deep venous system, the superficial system being most commonly involved compared to the deep venous system (outline in Table 11.1) [11]. The superficial system, especially the sagittal sinuses, has many sites of more turbulent blood flow. In addition, due to drainage of diploic, menin-geal, and emissary veins, it is more susceptible to infection-related clotting. The deep venous system has more extensive collateral circulation. Further, involvement of deep venous system is relatively difficult to recognize radiologically. The loca-tion of CSVT is age dependent (with older children having more lateral sinus involvement compared to neonates) and related to the etiology of thrombosis.

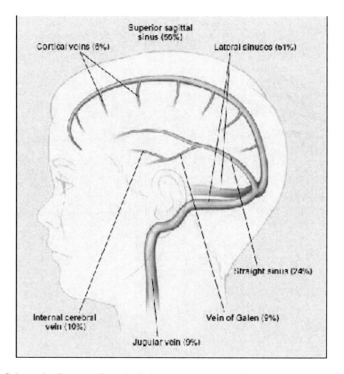

Fig. 11.1 Schematic diagram of cerebral sinus venous system. Numbers in parenthesis indicate the frequency of involvement. Patients may have multiple sites of involvement. Adopted from DeVeher G, Andrew M, Adam C, Bjorson B, Booth F, Buckley DJ et al. Cerebral sinovenous thrombosis in children New Eng. J. Med. 2001, 345: 417–23. Permission from New England Journal of Medicine

Etiology of CSVT in Children with Cancer

In pediatric age group, CSVT is usually a secondary phenomenon to an acute or chronic condition. Even in patients with chronic illness, acute risk factors are frequently observed. The common risk factors are outlined in Table 11.2.

The exact etiology of CSVT in children with cancer is not known but may be related to direct tumor invasion, therapy-induced (e.g., asparaginase) hypercoagulable state, or associated complications such as dehydration, infection, or a combination of the above factors [4, 5]. The risk of CSVT is shown to be increased by the presence of an underlying prothrombotic disorder [12, 13].

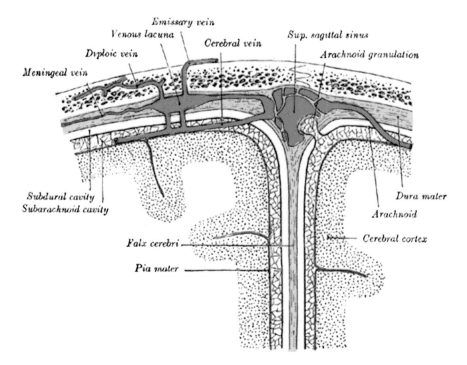

Fig. 11.2 Outline of cerebrospinal fluid circulation via arachnoid granulation. Emissary, diploic and meningeal veins drain into superficial venous sinuses. Adopted from Gray, Hendry. *Anatomy of the Human Body.* Philadelphia: Lea & Febiger, 1918; Bartleby.com, 2000. www.bartleby.com/107/ [Date of printout]. Permission from Bartleby.com to use figure

Table 11.1 Location of cerebral sinovenous thrombosis [2, 11]

Site	Involvement
Superficial	76–86%
Sagittal	
Lateral (sigmoid/transverse)	
Deep	14–38%
Straight	
Internal cerebral veins	
Vein of Galen	
Multiple	49%

Clinical Presentation

The clinical presentation depends on the age of the patients, associated risk factors, acuity of thrombosis, raised ICP, and location of thrombosis within the cerebral sinus system. The median duration is reported to be ~5 days with a range of 12 h–120 days [11]. Hence, a high index of suspicion is required.

Table 11.2 Risk factors predisposing older children to the development of CSVT

Acute systemic illness
Dehydration
Sepsis
Head and neck disorders
Prothrombotic states
Prothrombotic medications

Table 11.3 Neurologic signs and symptoms in children with CSVT

Seizures	58%
Generalized	26%
Focal	17%
Diffuse neurological signs	76%
Decreased level of consciousness	44%
Headache	34%
Papilledema	12%
Focal neurologic signs	42%
Hemiparesis	13%
Visual impairment	10%
Cranial nerve palsies	9%
Ataxia	4%
Speech impairment	4%
Sensory loss	2%
Other	16%

Infants and young children present with seizure (either focal or generalized) and lethargy, whereas older children present usually with signs of raised ICP (headache, vomiting, altered consciousness), seizure, or focal neurological signs (hemiparesis, cranial nerve palsy). Older patients may also present with signs of cavernous sinus syndrome. Signs and symptoms of associated underlying risk factors (e.g., dehydration, fever) may also be present. Although majority of patients with CSVT are symptomatic, in some patients, the CSVT could be asymptomatic and an incidental finding. Table 11.3 enlists the common clinical manifestation of CSVT.

Diagnosis of CSVT in Children

Please refer to Table 11.4 for advantages and disadvantages of various imaging modalities available for diagnosis of CSVT.

Principles of Management of CSVT

Current recommendations are derived from experience in adults. The mainstay of therapy is supportive care and anticoagulation therapy.

Table 11.4 Summary of available radiological imaging techniques for diagnosis of cerebral sinovenous thrombosis

Diagnostic modality	Radiological features	Advantages	Disadvantages
Head CT with contrast	Dense cord sign (1–5%) Empty delta sign (classic stigmata of CSVT) (10–30%)	Most commonly used Easy availability	Radiation exposure Limited sensitivity (68%) and specificity (52%) for diagnosis of adult CSVT
CT venogram	Delineates the venous system	Emerging as diagnostic tool for adults	High radiation exposure Rapid contrast injection rate
MRI	Delineates arterial, venous system as well as details brain structure	Noninvasive No radiation exposure Allows 3D visualization Better characterization of brain	Costly Requires sedation in younger children
MRI with MRV	Accurate visualization of cerebral sinuses and veins Improved sensitivity with addition of contrast study	Characterizes edema, infarction Unsuitable for very young infants	MRV may lead to false positive diagnosis of CSVT if the blood flow is slow Small children need sedation Require neuroradiologist for interpretation
Venous TCD	Emerging noninvasive diagnostic tool	Best suited for neonates	Not suitable for older children
Conventional angiogram	Characterization of vasculature	Gold standard for diagnosis of CSVT	Invasive Radiation exposure

CSVT cerebral sinovenous thrombosis, *CT* computerized tomography, *MRI* magnetic resonance imaging, *MRV* magnetic resonance venography, *TCD* transcranial Doppler study

Principles of Supportive Care

1. Treat underlying cause (e.g., infection, dehydration)
2. Management of raised ICP

Anticoagulation

Systemic anticoagulation therapy is reasonably safe and mostly effective. Proposed benefits include limitation of propagation of clot as well as prevention of formation of new thrombi.

Immediate anticoagulation is usually achieved through unfractionated heparin (UFH) or low-molecular-weight heparin (LMWH). Please refer to Chap. 10 for details of management of anticoagulation therapy.

Duration of Anticoagulation

The duration of anticoagulation therapy is usually 3–6 months. For more details, refer to Chap. 10.

Thrombolytic Therapy

Although there is no evidence regarding safety or efficacy of this modality, thrombolytic therapy has been increasingly used for management of CSVT. There is no data on pediatric patients except a few case reports. From adult studies, the thrombolytic therapy is limited to the following patients:

1. Patients who are comatose
2. Patients who have progressive neurological deterioration despite systemic anticoagulation
3. Absence of intracerebral hemorrhage prior to the start of therapy.
   In pediatric oncology, we rarely need to resort to such invasive therapy.

Outcome of Patients with CSVT

This information is based on observational studies conducted in neonates and general pediatric population.

1. High mortality (8–16%)
2. Long-term neurological morbidity (22–38%) including motor deficit, neuropsychiatric dysfunction, visual impairment, pseudotumor cerebri, seizure, and headache
3. Recurrent CSVT in ~2–8% of children

References

1. Raffini L, Huang Y-S, Witmer C, Feudtner C. A significant increase in venous thromboembolism in U.S. Children's Hospitals from 2001–2007. J Thromb Haemost 2009;7(2).
2. DeVeber G, Andrew M, Adam C, Bjorson B, Booth F, Buckley DJ et al. Cerebral sinovenous thrombosis in children New Eng J Med 2001, 345: 417–423
3. Raizer JJ, DeAngelis LM. Cerebral sinus thrombosis diagnosed by MRI and MR venography in cancer patients. Neurology 2000; 54:1222–1226
4. Wermes C, Prondzinski M vD, Lichtinghagen R, Barthels M, Welte K, Sykora KW. Clinical relevance of genetic risk factors for thrombosis in pediatric oncology patients with central venous catheters. Eur J Pediatr 1999; 158 (Suppl3): S143–S146

5. Packer RJ, Rorke LB, Lange BJ, Siegel KR, Evans AE. Cerebrovascular accidents in children with cancer. Pediatrics 1985; 76:194–201

6. Athale UH, Chan AKC. Thrombosis in children with acute lymphoblastic leukemia Part I: Epidemiology of thrombosis in children with acute lymphoblastic leukemia. Thrombosis Research 2003; 111: 125–131

7. Mitchell LG, Sutor AN, Andrew M. Hemostasis in childhood acute lymphoblastic leukemia: coagulopathy induced by disease and treatment. Seminars in Thrombosis & Hemostasis, 1995; 21:390–401

8. Caruso V, Lacoviello L, Castelnuovo AD, Storti S, Mariani G, Gaetano GD, Donati MB. Thrombotic complications in childhood acute lymphoblastic leukemia: a meta-analysis of 17 prospective studies comprising 1752 patients. Blood, 2006; 108:2216–2222

9. Reddingius RE, Patte C, Couanet D, Kalifa C, Lemerle J. Dural sinus thrombosis in children with cancer. Med Ped Oncol 1997, 29:296–302

10. Legrand I, Lalande G, Neuenschwander S, Dulac O, Kalifa LG. Thrombosis du sinus longitudinal superior au cours du treatment de lymphoma hez l'enfant. J Radiol 1986; 67:595–600

11. Carpenter J, Tsuchida T. Cerebral sinovenous thrombosis in children. Current neurology and Neuroscience reports 2007;7:139–146

12. Kenet G, Lutkhoff LK, Albisetti M, Bernard T, Bonduel M, et al. Impact of thrombophilia on risk of arterial ischemic stroke and cerebral sinovenous thrombosis: a systematic review and meta-analysis of observational studies. Circulation 2010; 121: 1838–1847

13. Trenor CC, Michelson AD. Editorial: Thrombophilia and pediatric stroke. Circulation 2010; 121:1795–1797

Chapter 12
Central Venous Line-related Thrombosis

Uma Athale and Anthony Chan

Keywords Accidental dislodgments • Ball-valve clots • Central venous lines • Compressibility • CVL dysfunction • CVL occlusion • CVL-related thrombosis • Mural thrombosis • Pinch-off syndrome • Port-A-Cath • Postthrombotic syndrome • Prothrombotic effects • Sleeve thrombus • Thrombolytic agents • Venogram

Long-term central venous lines (CVL) have improved the quality of care and quality of life of children with cancer. The CVLs are commonly used to deliver chemotherapy, blood products, parenteral nutrition, and other intravenous therapy as well as to facilitate repeated blood drawing essential for the monitoring of these patients [1]. Hence, the use of CVL has become standard of care for venous access in children with malignancy.

Types of CVL: Two types of CVLs commonly used in children with cancer:

1. Internal CVL: subcutaneous venous access port or totally implantable venous access device (e.g., Port-A-Cath or Mediport).
2. External CVL: could be tunneled (e.g., Hickman, Broviac, or Groshong) catheters or peripherally inserted central catheters (PICC). The external CVLs can be with or without valves.

Each of these lines could be single- or multi-lumen; choice of the CVL depends on the age and the need of the patient.

U. Athale (✉) • A. Chan
Division of Hematology/Oncology, McMaster Children's Hospital,
Hamilton, ON, Canada L8S 4K1
e-mail: athaleu@mcmaster.ca

K. Scheinemann and A.E. Boyce (eds.), *Emergencies in Pediatric Oncology*,
DOI 10.1007/978-1-4614-1174-1_12, © Springer Science+Business Media, LLC 2012

Complications of CVL

CVLs are associated with early complications, mostly surgical, related to the line insertion (e.g., bleeding and pneumothorax) and late complications, mostly medical (e.g., infection and thrombosis) [1–4]. Two recent studies have identified a CVL-related complication rate of 40–46% [1, 5]. Infection and thromboembolism (TE) are the most common and serious medical complications associated with CVL. Yet another common, but less studied, complication is CVL occlusion (also known as CVL dysfunction, blockage, or malfunction) [5–7]. In this chapter, we will discuss the two common complications of CVL, namely CVL occlusion and CVL-related thromboembolism.

CVL Occlusion

Occlusion is usually defined as inability to infuse fluids or withdraw blood [2, 5, 7]. The occlusion could be partial when there is difficulty either in aspiration or infusion, or complete when there is difficulty in both aspiration and infusion. The occlusion can be acute or gradual.

The occlusion may result from mechanical and/or nonmechanical causes. Mechanical causes include kinking, dislodgment, fracture, and leakage, whereas nonmechanical causes include thrombosis, intraluminal precipitation due to medication or total parenteral nutrition (TPN) [2, 3]. About one third of patients would have CVL occlusion within 1–2 years of catheter placement, and about one third of occluded CVLs need to be removed [2, 3, 8, 9]. Further, occluded CVLs result in interruption or delay of the chemotherapy which may affect outcome. Hence, an early and accurate diagnosis of etiology of CVL occlusion is important for effective management and prevention of complications. Table 12.1 outlines the common causes of CVL occlusion.

Nonthrombotic Causes of CVL Dysfunction/Occlusion

The causes of mechanical problems are variable depending upon the type of CVL, vein of access, and method of CVL insertion (cutdown vs venipuncture) as well as CVL tip positioning. The common mechanical problems associated with external lines are accidental dislodgments (reported to be as high as 24%) and damage to the external part of the CVL. One study observed that over 40% of CVL dysfunctions were nonthrombotic [10].

Table 12.1 lists the various mechanical problems and the diagnosis and management of the same. A common problem is that the CVL tip is too close to the vessel wall or it is blocked by the endothelium leading to "positional" functioning of the CVL.

Table 12.1 Etiology, diagnosis, and management of CVL occlusion

Causes	Diagnosis	Management
Mechanical causes		
Kink in the CVL, tight suture or clamp	Inspection of the CVL system	Treat the cause
Port (Huber) needle displacement or rupture of the port septum	Inspection, dye study	Treat the cause
Malposition of CVL tip or CVL migration	Chest X-ray	Guide wire manipulation or surgical repositioning
Displacement or dislodgment of CVL	Chest X-ray, linogram or dye study, ECHO	Surgical repair, repositioning, or replacement
Fracture of the catheter, rupture of port septum	Swelling surrounding the port or leakage from the catheter, chest X-ray, linogram or dye study	Repair or replacement
Pinch-off syndrome	Chest X-ray, fluoroscopy	Remove and replace catheter if at risk of fracture
Non-mechanical causes		
Medication- or TPN-related Calcium phosphate precipitate, lipid emulsion	Review the infusates and medication Check compatibility	Adjust the pH and compatibility of solutions. Consider chemical lysis of the precipitate with instillation of acidic or basic solution or ethanol
Thrombotic causes		
Fibrin sheath	Linogram or dye study, ECHO	Local thrombolytic instillation, guide wire-guided removal
Intraluminal or CVL tip clot	Linogram or dye study	Local thrombolytic instillation, guide wire-guided removal
Mural or right atrial thrombosis	Linogram or dye study, ECHO	Systemic anticoagulation, surgical thrombectomy if indicated
CVL-related DVT	Linogram or dye study, ECHO, bilateral venography, Doppler ultrasonography, MRV	Systemic anticoagulation, CVL removal if indicated

CVL central venous line, *ECHO* echocardiogram, *DVT* deep venous thrombosis, *MRV* magnetic resonance venogram

Repositioning maneuvers like raising the ipsilateral arm, sitting up, standing, rolling over, or bending forward or coughing may improve "positional" functioning. A rare but potentially fatal problem is the "pinch-off syndrome" as shown in Fig. 12.1. The "pinch-off syndrome" occurs in ~ 1% of CVLs but may result in ~ 40% of catheter fractures with subsequent embolization through heart to pulmonary vasculature [3, 11].

Inappropriate composition of TPN or drugs or incompatible solutions may result in precipitation within the CVL lumen and "chemical" blockage. For example, inappropriate concentrations of calcium and phosphorus may lead to precipitation of

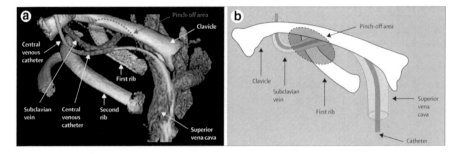

Fig. 12.1 The "pinch off" area is the narrow angle between the first rib and the lateral portion of the clavicle. CVL passing through this area is at risk for compression or fragmentation. Panel a is a 3-dimensional CT image which shows a CVL passing externally parallel to the subclavian vein before inserting into the superior vena cava. Panel b shows a CVL which is internal in the subclavian vein while passing through the pinch off area. The CVL external to the subclavian vein while passing through the "pinch off" area as shown in Panel a is at higher risk of "pinch-off syndrome" and fracture. Adopted from Baskin JL, Pii C-H, Reiss U, Wilimas J, Metzger M, Ribiero R, Howard SC. Management of Occlusion and thrombosis associated with long-term indwelling central venous catheters. Lancet 2009; 374: 159-69. Permission given from Lancet

calcium phosphate crystals especially if the pH of the solution is high, or drugs with high pH (e.g., phenytoin) may precipitate in acidic solutions. These kinds of occlusions could be treated with appropriate flush solutions, e.g., alkaline solutions like sodium bicarbonate (1.0 mol/L) or sodium hydroxide (0.1 mol/L) for acidic precipitates or acidic solutions like hydrochloric acid (0.1 mol/L) for basic precipitates. Blockage resulting from lipid emulsions of TPN may be dissolved with 70% ethanol [3, 8, 9]. However, these solutions (especially hydrochloric acid) can cause damage to the catheter wall and may lead to other side effects (e.g., dizziness with alcohol) and hence are not widely used [3].

Thrombotic CVL Occlusion

Thrombotic occlusion is the most common cause of CVL dysfunction [4–6, 8]. This can result from:

1. Sleeve thrombus: This is a fibrin sheath surrounding the catheter and is the most common type of thrombotic occlusion. The fibrin sheath may develop soon after CVL placement but usually within 2 weeks. The fibrin sheath usually does not affect CVL function but may result in partial obstruction which is pressure dependent.
2. Clots at the catheter tip (ball-valve clots): These are the clots developing on the external surface of the CVL and may block the tip of the line.
3. Intraluminal clots: These are clots developing within the lumen of the CVL and account for ~ 5–25% of all CVL occlusions.

4. Mural thrombosis: This is the formation of nonocclusive thrombus in the catheterized vessel that adheres to the vessel wall and can occlude the tip of the catheter.
5. Occlusive deep venous thrombosis (DVT) of the catheterized vessel with or without involvement of central vasculature.

The sleeve thrombus or the ball-valve clots may result in partial obstruction by creating one-way flow and usually result in withdrawal obstruction. While aspirating for blood, the negative pressure creates a ball-valve effect by pulling the fibrin sheath or CVL tip clot which occludes the flow in the lumen. This blockage resolves when the pressure of infusion or flushing pushes the fibrin sheath or a small clot away from the tip.

Evaluation and Management of Patients with Thrombotic CVL Occlusion

Table 12.1 outlines the diagnosis and management of various causes of CVL occlusion. Figure 12.2 describes the algorithm of evaluation and management of CVL occlusion.

Various thrombolytic agents are usually used empirically to treat suspected thrombotic occlusion. Table 12.2 describes commonly used thrombolytic agents. The recommended approach includes delivery of a thrombolytic agent into the CVL lumen with a dwell time of at least 30 min. Repeat the dose if necessary. However, if after the second dose the patency is not restored, then further studies are warranted to rule out occlusive DVT.

CVL-Related Thrombosis

Presence of CVL is the single-most important risk factor for development of thrombosis in children [4]. This risk is further exaggerated in children with cancer due to the prothrombotic effects of cancer and the chemotherapy. Majority of CVL-related thromboses occur in upper extremities since most long-term CVLs are placed in the upper venous system. These CVL-related thrombosis could be symptomatic (with pain, tenderness to palpation, edema, skin discoloration, warmth, and dilated veins) or asymptomatic [12]. About 12% of children with CVL are reported to have symptomatic CVL-related thrombosis whereas up to 50% have asymptomatic CVL-related thrombosis. The presence of symptoms reflects the site of obstruction and acuteness of obstruction as well as the methods of diagnosis or screening. In children, especially younger age group, the symptoms of TE are difficult to detect, and hence, even significant TE may go undiagnosed. Hence, a high index of suspicion is necessary. Table 12.3 lists the proposed risk factors predisposing to CVL-related thrombosis.

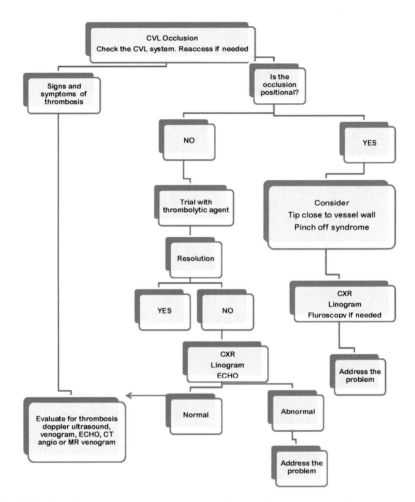

Fig. 12.2 Algorithm outlining the commonly used steps for evaluation and management of patients with CVL occlusion. When faced with an occluded line, please check the CVL system and rule out any local issues like pinching of external tubing. Consider re-accessing the port. Systematic evaluation for signs and symptom of thrombosis is essential. CVL=central venous line, CXR=chest X-ray, ECHO=echocardiography, CT=computerized tomography, MR=magnetic resonance

Complications of CVL-Related Thrombosis [2,4,12–15]

1. Pulmonary embolism (PE): potentially fatal complication. About 16% of children with CVL-related thrombosis developed PE, 3% with fatal PE.
2. Increased risk of infection: Proteins within the thrombus, such as fibrinogen and fibronectin, enhance the adherence of microorganisms such as staphylococci, resulting in CVL-related bloodstream infection.
3. CVL dysfunction: due to the blockage of the CVL tip.

Table 12.2 Summary of thrombolytic agents used for restoration of patency of blocked CVL

Agent	Source	Recommended dwell time	Efficacy for CVL clearance [2]	Advantages/disadvantages
Alteplase	Tissue plasminogen activator produced by recombinant DNA from vascular epithelium	30–120 min	50% after 1st dose and 86% after 2nd dose	Safe and effective High cost
Reteplase	Recombinant modified variant of human tPA produced from *E. coli*	30–60 min	70% after 1st dose and 95% after 2nd dose	Longer half-life than alteplase. Lower affinity to fibrin resulting in better penetration of the clot
Recombinant urokinase	Recombinant urokinase produced by transfected mammalian cells	15–30 min	60% after 1st dose and 80% after 2nd dose	Rapid restoration of patency 0.6–1.8% risk of major bleeding Restricted access

Table 12.3 Proposed risk factors for development of CVL-related thrombosis

Type of CVL	Internal lines (e.g., Port-A-Cath) are at higher risk of developing thrombosis than external lines (e.g., Hickman)
Duration of CVL	Longer duration of CVL dwell increases the risk
Multiple CVLs	Increase the risk of thrombosis
CVL insertion technique	CVLs inserted via venipuncture have increased risk of thrombosis compared to those inserted by venous cutdown
Site of insertion	CVLs located in left subclavian are at increased risk of thrombosis than those in right subclavian
Infection	Prior CVL infections are shown to increase the risk of thrombosis
Type of underlying malignancy	Patients with acute lymphoblastic leukemia or patients with mediastinal mass are shown to have higher risk of thrombosis
CVL dysfunction	Dysfunctional CVLs have increased association of thrombosis

4. Postthrombotic syndrome (PTS): long-term complication resulting in edema, skin discoloration, pain, and, in severe cases, skin ulceration. Significant PTS is reported in ~10–20% of children with CVL-related thrombosis.
5. Recurrent thrombosis: occurs in ~7–8% of children.

Diagnosis of CVL-Related Thrombosis [3, 12, 16, 17]

Because of the non-invasiveness and ease of performance, ultrasound (US) plus doppler is the preferred method for diagnosis of TE in children. The most reliable diagnostic criterion for thrombosis by US is noncompressibility of the vein.

Table 12.4 Summary of pros and cons of various imaging modalities for diagnosis of CVL-related DVT

Imaging modality	Advantages	Disadvantages
Doppler ultrasound	Noninvasive, easy access, cheap, and accurate for diagnosis of jugular vein and lower extremity DVT	Due to poor sensitivity, unsuitable for diagnosis of thrombosis in vessels within the thoracic cavity
Venogram	Current gold standard for diagnosis with ~ 80% sensitivity	Invasive test with exposure to contrast dye and radiation, small children may require sedation
CT venogram	Three-dimensional reconstruction improves the diagnostic accuracy	Radiation exposure, small children may require sedation
MR venogram	No radiation exposure	Motion artifact may make interpretation difficult, high cost, sedation needed for small children

CVL central venous line, *DVT* deep venous thrombosis, *CT* computerized tomography, *MR* magnetic resonance

A solid material like a blood clot inside the lumen of a vessel prevents the vessel from being compressed with pressure. Thus, compressibility of the vessel rules out DVT on US. Other findings like intraluminal echogenicity or absence of doppler flow on US are relatively nonspecific and lack sensitivity. Although compression US is the diagnostic test of choice for suspected lower venous system deep venous thrombosis (DVT), it is not a sensitive technique for the diagnosis of DVT in upper venous system (central subclavian vein, brachiocephalic vein, and superior vena cava). Within the thoracic cage, the noncompressibility of the vessel cannot be assessed due to the presence of ribs [16]. Hence, bilateral venogram is considered to be a gold standard for the diagnosis of DVT of the central vasculature. However, US is a reliable method for evaluation of jugular veins. Table 12.4 describes the advantages and disadvantages of various imaging techniques available for diagnosis of CVL-related DVT. In patients with suspected CVL-related DVT, we start with doppler ultrasound first. If negative and clinical suspicion is very strong, we proceed with venography. Sometimes other noninvasive tests like echocardiography may also be helpful to diagnose DVT. However, one may still like to have a venogram to define the extent of the clot and monitor the effects of anticoagulation.

Management of CVL-Related Thrombosis

The aims of management are reduction in acute morbidity and mortality and prevention or reduction of late complications. However, optimal management is controversial. The management is mainly dictated by the continued need for CVL. Figure 12.3 outlines the management of CVL-related thrombosis [18].

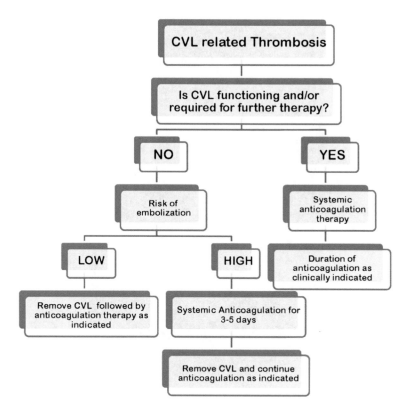

Fig. 12.3 Principles of management of CVL-related deep venous thrombosis. If a CVL is not functional or not required, it should be removed. Anticoagulation therapy with low molecular weight heparin (LMWH) is usually a preferred mode of therapy in children with cancer. In absence of standard guidelines, the duration of anticoagulation therapy is usually an individualized decision based on the need for continued use of the CVL, size of the clot and underlying prothrombotic condition. Usual duration of LMWH is 6–12 weeks after the CVL is removed. If the CVL remains *in situ,* the patient may continue prophylactic doses of LMWH after initial 6–12 weeks of anticoagulation therapy. Please refer to Chapter 11 for further details. CVL=Central venous line

Case 1

A 4-year-and-10-month-old girl underwent Port-A-Cath insertion for newly diagnosed ALL. There were ongoing issues with flushes and blood return, but there was no swelling or pain. Patient underwent linogram which demonstrated leakage of the contrast at the junction of the reservoir and the catheter. Patient underwent immediate port revision (Fig. 12.4).

Case 2

Eight year old girl with standard risk acute lymphoblastic leukemia (ALL), on maintenance therapy on Dana-Farber Cancer Institute ALL Consortium protocol was noted to have dilated veins on upper chest and abdomen. Her port-a-cath had difficulties in bleeding back although it flushed well. She underwent two linograms

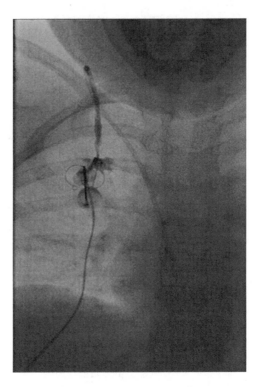

Fig. 12.4 Linogram showing leakage around the port connection

5 months apart (Fig. 12.5a and 12.5b) which were normal. Finally she underwent a venogram which confirmed an occlusive right subclavian and axillary vein thrombosis with extensive collateral veins (Fig. 12.5c).

Case 3
Seventeen year old patient was receiving chemotherapy for high risk ALL. At the time of diagnosis she received a peripherally inserted central catheter (PICC) which was later changed to port-a-cath in right jugular vein. She and her friends noted increasing prominence of chest veins especially on right side. There was no pain, tenderness or other problems. Her port has problems withdrawing blood back but otherwise infused well. She underwent an ultarsonography of upper venous system in July 2009 which reported patency of axillary, subclavian, basilic and jugular veins and did not detect any deep venous thrombosis. Bilateral venogram performed in August 2009 detected complete obstruction of the right subclavian vein from the level of first rib till innominate vein with extensive collateral formation. Collaterals were seen to ipsilateral jugular vein and contralateral brachiocephalic vein (Fig. 12.6a and 12.6b). Left sided arm veins were widely patent (Fig. 12.6c).

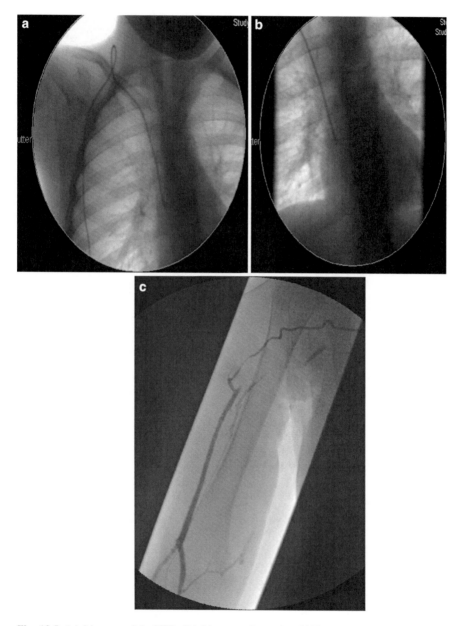

Fig. 12.5 (a) Linogram July 2005. (b) Linogram December 2005. (c) Venogram right upper venous system (December 2005)

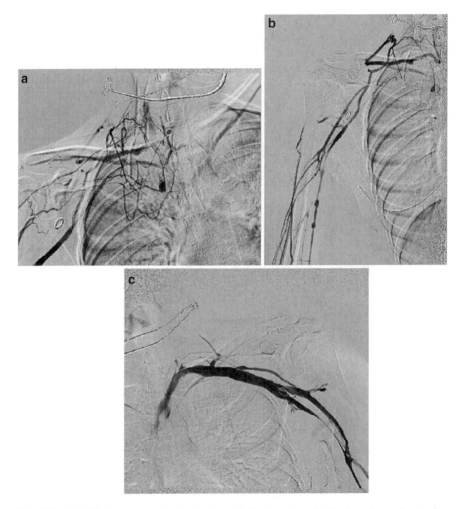

Fig. 12.6 (**a, b**) Right arm venography showing subclavian vein occlusive thrombus and extensive collateral veins. **c**) Left arm venography showing widely open veins

References

1. Fratino G, Molinari AC, Parodi S, Longo S, Saracco P, Castagnola E, Haupt R. Central venous catheter-related complications in children with oncological/hematological diseases: an observational study of 418 devices. Annals of Oncology 2005; 16:648–54

2. Baskin JL, Pui C-H, Reiss U, Wilimas J, Metzger M, Ribiero R, Howard SC. Management of occlusion and thrombosis associated with long-term indwelling central venous catheters. Lancet 2009; 374:159–69

3. Male C, Chait P, Andrew M, Hanna K, Julian J, Mitchell L, PARKAA investigators. Central venous line related-thrombosis: association with central venous line location and insertion technique. Blood 2003; 101:4273–8

4. Massicotte MP, Dix D, Monagle P, Adams M, Andrew M. Central venous catheter related thrombosis in children: analysis of the Canadian registry of venous thromboembolic complications. J Pediatr 1998; 133:770–6

5. Journeycake JM, Buchanan GR. Catheter-related deep venous thrombosis and other catheter complications in children with cancer. J Clin Oncol 2006; 24;4575–80

6. Athale UH, Siciliano S, Thabane L, Pai N, Cox S, Lathia A, Khan AA, Armstrong A, Chan AKC. Epidemiology and clinical risk factors predisposing to thromboembolism in children with cancer. Pediatric Blood and Cancer, 2008, 51:792–7

7. Deitcher SR, Gajjar A, Kun L, Heideman RL. Clinically evident venous thromboembolic events in children with brain tumors. Journal of Pediatrics 2004; 145:848–50

8. Lokich JJ, Bothe A, Benotti P, Moore C. Complications and management of implanted venous access catheters. J Clin Oncology 1985; 3:710–17

9. Moore C, Strong D, Childress J, Fougere B, Gotthardt S. Surveillance of the patient receiving infusional cancer chemotherapy: nursing role in recognition and management of catheter-related complications. J Infusional Chemotherapy 1996; 6:171–180

10. Stephens LC, Haire WD, Kotulak GD. Are clinical signs accurate indicators of the cause of central venous catheter occlusion? J Parenter Enteral Nutr 1995;19;75–9

11. Fazeny-Dorner B, Wenzel C, Berlanovich A, Sunder-Plassmann G, Grenix H, Marosi C, Muhm M. Central venous catheter pinch off and fracture: recognition, prevention and management. Bone Marrow Transplantation 2003;31:927–30

12. Mitchell LG, Andrew M, Hanna K, et al. A prospective cohort study determining the prevalence of thrombotic events in children with acute lymphoblastic leukemia and a central venous line who are treated with L-asparaginase. Results of the Prophylactic Antithrombin Replacement in Kids with Acute Lymphoblastic Leukemia Treated with Asparaginase (PARKAA) study. Cancer. 2003; 97:508–16.

13. Rosovsky RP, Kuter DJ. Catheter-related thrombosis in cancer patients: pathophysiology, diagnosis and management. Hematol Oncol Clin N Am 2005; 19:183–202

14. Ruud E, Holmstrome H, Hopp E, Wesenberg F. Central line-associated venous late effects in children without prior history of thrombosis. Acta Paediatrica 2006, 95:1060–5

15. Cesaro C, Corro R, Pelocin A et al. A prospective survey on incidence and outcome of Broviac/Hickman catheter-related complications in pediatric patients affected by hematological ad oncological diseases. Ann Hematol 2004; 83:183–8

16. Prandoni P, Bernardi E. Upper extremity deep venous thrombosis. Current Opinion Pulmonary Medicine 1999; 5:222

17. Chunilal SD, Ginsberg JS. Advances in the diagnosis of venous thromboembolism: a multimodal approach. J Thrombosis and Thrombolysis 2001; 12:53–7

18. Monagle P, Chalmers E, Chan AKC et al. Antithrombotic therapy in neonates and children: American College of Chest Physicians evidence-based clinical practice guidelines (8th edition) Chest 2008; 133:887–968

Chapter 13
Chemotherapeutic Drugs

Paula MacDonald

Keywords Asparaginase • Cell cycle • Chemotherapeutic agents • Cross sensitivity
• Cytotoxic spill • Decontamination • Desensitization protocols • Extravasation •
Glucarpidase • Hypersensitivity reactions • Leucovorin • Methotrexate • Necrotic
tissue • Personal protective equipment • Renal clearance

Introduction

The goal of chemotherapy in the treatment of cancer is to kill malignant cells and
prevent metastases. Cancer cells have a rapid rate of cellular division; therefore, chemotherapeutic agents are designed to destroy these rapidly dividing cells. It is important to understand the mechanism of action of the various classes of chemotherapy
drugs as therapeutic protocols often use multiple drugs that may have synergistic or
enhanced effect against malignant cells when used in combination. Knowledge of
how these drugs work is also important in predicting potential toxic effects, thus
allowing for the development of chemotherapy regimens that minimize the risk of
severe toxicity through the combination of agents with different side effect profiles.

Classes of Chemotherapeutic Drugs

Chemotherapeutic agents can be divided into several classes based on mechanism
of action, chemical structure, biologic source, or effect on the cell cycle. These agents
were formerly classified on the basis of where they act in the cell cycle. Cell cycle-
specific drugs act only on a specific stage of the cell cycle (e.g., methotrexate affects

P. MacDonald (✉)
Division of Hematology/Oncology, McMaster Children's Hospital,
1200 Main Street West, Hamilton, ON, Canada L8N 3Z5
e-mail: macdonap@hhsc.ca

K. Scheinemann and A.E. Boyce (eds.), *Emergencies in Pediatric Oncology*,
DOI 10.1007/978-1-4614-1174-1_13, © Springer Science+Business Media, LLC 2012

cells during DNA synthesis or S phase), while cell cycle-nonspecific chemotherapy drugs affect cells during all stages of the cell cycle, including resting cells. However, there are too many exceptions to this classification. A more useful means of classifying these agents is on the basis of their mechanism of action and derivation [1]. Table 13.1 describes the various categories of chemotherapeutic agents.

Table 13.1 Classification of chemotherapeutic agents [1, 2]

Classification	Mechanism of action	Common toxicities	Agents
Alkylating agents	Interfere with DNA replication and transcription by cross-linking DNA strands, causing DNA strand breakage and abnormal base pairing Most active against cancer cells in G0 (resting) phase (ref 1)	*Myelosuppression Other common toxicities: nausea, vomiting, alopecia, reduced fertility, secondary malignancies Nephrotoxicity (cisplatin, cyclophosphamide, ifosfamide) Ototoxicity, neurotoxicity (cisplatin, carboplatin, oxaliplatin) Hemorrhagic cystitis (cyclophosphamide, ifosfamide)	Busulfan Carmustine(BCNU) Carboplatin Cisplatin Chlorambucil Cyclophosphamide Dacarbazine (DTIC) Ifosfamide Lomustine(CCNU) Mechlorethamine Melphalan Oxaliplatin Procarbazine Temozolomide Thiotepa
Antimetabolites	Structural analogues of nucleotide bases that interfere with synthesis of protein, DNA, and RNA in the cell (ref 1)	*Myelosuppression *Gastrointestinal mucositis (including stomatitis, diarrhea) Other common toxicities: nausea, vomiting elevated transaminases (methotrexate) conjunctivitis (high-dose Ara-C)	Folic acid antagonists Methotrexate Pyrimidine antagonists 5-Azacytidine 5-Fluorouracil Cytosine arabinoside (Ara-C) Gemcitabine Purine antagonists 6-Mercaptopurine 6-Thioguanine Fludarabine Cladribine
Antitumor antibiotics	Covalently bind DNA; interfere with RNA transcription and DNA replication Anthracyclines also associated with free radical formation and inhibition of topoisomerase II enzyme	*Myelosuppression *Cardiomyopathy(cumulative effect with anthracyclines) Other common toxicities: oral mucositis, alopecia, nausea, vomiting, secondary malignancies, hepatoxicity, radiation recall *Interstitial pulmonary fibrosis and skin hyperpigmentation (bleomycin)	Anthracyclines Daunorubicin Doxorubicin Idarubicin Mitoxantrone Bleomycin Dactinomycin Mitomycin-C

(continued)

Table 13.1 (continued)

Classification	Mechanism of action	Common toxicities	Agents
Topoisomerase I inhibitors	Inhibit DNA and RNA synthesis by preventing the unwinding of DNA strands (via inhibition of the enzyme topoisomerase I)	***Myelosuppression** Other common toxicities: nausea, vomiting, alopecia ***Diarrhea (irinotecan)** secondary malignancies	Camptothecin Irinotecan Topotecan (*These agents could also be classified as alkylating agents)
Plant alkaloids	Vinca alkaloids inhibit mitotic spindle formation by binding to tubulin (arrest cells in metaphase) Epipodophyllotoxins inhibit topoisomerase II enzyme and produce DNA strand breaks Taxanes bind to microtubules and inhibit their disassembly; M phase–specific	***Myelosuppression** (vinblastine, vinorelbine, etoposide, teniposide, taxanes) ***Peripheral neuropathy** (vincristine, paclitaxel) Other common toxicities: nausea, vomiting, alopecia, hypotension (with rapid etoposide infusion), constipation, jaw pain (vincristine)	*Vinca alkaloids* Vinorelbine Vinblastine Vincristine *Epipodophyllotoxins* Etoposide (VP-16) Teniposide (VM-26) *Taxanes* Docetaxel Paclitaxel
Corticosteroids	Exact mechanism not fully understood. Steroids appear to form a complex with macromolecules in the cytoplasm of the cell, which binds with DNA and modifies the transcription process. (ref 1) Direct lytic action in leukemia and lymphoma cells	Acne Cushingoid appearance Fluid/sodium retention Gastric ulcers, reflux (give with food) Hyperglycemia Hyperphagia Hypertension Immunosuppression Insomnia Personality/mood changes Pituitary–adrenal suppression Osteopenia/osteoporosis ***Avascular necrosis**	Dexamethasone Hydrocortisone Methylprednisolone Prednisone
Miscellaneous agents	Hydroxyurea interferes with ribonucleotide reductase enzyme and inhibits DNA synthesis L-Asparaginase (enzyme) hydrolyzes serum asparagine to aspartic acid and ammonia, depleting asparagine and inhibiting protein synthesis in leukemia cells	Hydroxyurea: ***Myelosuppression** nausea, vomiting, diarrhea L-Asparaginase: ***Hypersensitivity reactions** (including urticaria, angioedema, bronchospasm, hypotension), hyperglycemia, thrombosis, acute pancreatitis	Hydroxyurea L-Asparaginase (derived from *Escherichia coli* or *Erwinia* bacteria) PEG-L-Asparaginase (coated with polyethylene glycol to reduce immunogenicity)

* A dose-limiting toxicity

Table 13.2 Biological therapies for cancer [1, 4, 5]

Targeted therapies	e.g., Imatinib mesylate, gefitinib, bortezomib
Designed to attack cancer cells with mutated versions of certain genes or cells overexpressing copies of a specific gene	Imatinib mesylate is a protein tyrosine kinase inhibitor that selectively inhibits the growth of leukemia cells expressing the Bcr-Abl fusion protein. It has been combined with standard chemotherapy agents for the treatment of Philadelphia chromosome–positive acute lymphoblastic leukemia (ALL) in pediatric patients
Differentiating agents	e.g., Tretinoin (all-trans retinoic acid, ATRA) has proven effective in the treatment of acute promyelocytic leukemia (APL)
The retinoids are naturally occurring analogues of vitamin A that induce tumor cell differentiation and maturation, leading to apoptosis	cis-retinoic acid (isotretinoin) is used post consolidation therapy for stage IV neuroblastoma to treat minimal residual disease.
Common side effects of the retinoids include dry skin and mucosa, photosensitivity, and elevated serum triglyceride levels	It reduces proliferation of neuroblastoma cells and decreases expression of the MYCN oncogene
Antiangiogenic agents	Thalidomide is a direct inhibitor of endothelial cells and therefore inhibits vascular endothelial growth factor (VEGF)-stimulated angiogenesis. It has demonstrated antitumor activities in a number of cancers, especially high-grade gliomas and multiple myeloma. Major dose-limiting side effect is sedation. Published experience in children is limited
New classification of drugs designed to limit further tumor growth and development of metastases by returning proliferating microvessels associated with malignant tissue to their normal resting state and preventing their regrowth	
Biotherapy (immunotherapy)	Interleukin-2 (IL-2) increases the activity of lymphocytes, primarily killer T-cells[6], and is used to treat neuroblastoma
Use of biologically derived agents to activate the immune system to more effectively recognize and attack cancer cells[4, 6]	
Active immunotherapies stimulate the body's own immune system to fight cancer and include interferons, interleukins, and cancer vaccines	Rituximab, alemtuzumab, gemtuzumab, and trastuzumab are a few monoclonal antibodies incorporated into current treatment regimens
Passive immunotherapies (i.e., monoclonal antibodies) stimulate cell kill by targeting proteins on the surface of cancer cells, thus marking the cells for destruction by the immune system. They can also target chemotherapy or radioactive isotopes to the cancer cells directly or block receptors that receive growth signals	CH 14.18 antibody is a chimeric (murine–human) antibody specific for the GD2 ganglioside expressed on neuroblastoma cells. It kills the cells by complement activation and antibody-dependent cellular cytotoxicity. Use of this agent has been limited by its toxicity profile which includes capillary leak syndrome, hypotension, infusion-related reactions, neuropathic pain, myelosuppression, and arrhythmias

There are other agents and biological treatments used to treat cancer that are not classified as chemotherapy [3]. These agents have been designed to target specific malignant cells rather than normal, healthy cells and often have less serious side effects than chemotherapeutic agents (Table 13.2).

Methotrexate Clearance and Toxicity

Methotrexate (MTX), a folic acid antagonist, competes with dihydrofolate to bind to the enzyme, dihydrofolate reductase (DHFR). This leads to inhibition of tetrahydrofolate synthesis and a reduction in intracellular reduced folates. Once the pools of reduced folates are depleted, DNA synthesis stops, and the result is serious toxicity to both tumor cells and normal cells within the body [1].

Methotrexate undergoes hepatic metabolism, but the primary route of elimination during the first 24 h is renal excretion of the unmetabolized drug [6]. Renal clearance of MTX involves glomerular filtration, active tubular secretion, and tubular reabsorption [6, 7]. Reduced renal function results in an increased elimination half-life of MTX and predisposes the patient to adverse effects, such as mucositis, pancytopenia, gastrointestinal desquamation, and hepatotoxicity [6]. Methotrexate can also accumulate in body cavities and fluid collections, such as ascites and pleural effusions, from which it will slowly redistribute [1]. This release from "third space" fluid collections can lead to excessive toxicity. Drainage of such collections is recommended prior to MTX administration when possible [8].

High doses of MTX (i.e., 1–20 g/m^2) in treatment protocols for lymphoma, leukemia, and osteogenic sarcoma have the potential to cause severe and potentially fatal toxicities. Patients receiving such doses require routine monitoring of serum creatinine and plasma MTX concentrations following administration [1]. High-dose methotrexate (HDMTX) produces MTX concentrations in the urine above the solubility index at a pH <7. This may result in precipitation of MTX and its metabolites in the acidic urine, causing obstruction of the kidney tubules. Tubular injury could lead to HDMTX-induced acute renal failure, which is a medical emergency. Adequate hydration (intravenous fluids at 125 mL/m^2/h) and urine alkalinization (urine pH $\geq$7 and $\leq$8) with sodium bicarbonate are required with HDMTX to prevent renal toxicity [1, 6, 9].

Leucovorin (folinic acid) administration is also required to prevent severe toxicity with MTX doses greater than or equal to 500 mg/m^2 [8, 9]. Leucovorin is a derivative of tetrahydrofolic acid (i.e., a reduced folate) that can rescue normal cells from the toxicity of HDMTX by replenishing these cells with an alternative source of reduced folate for DNA synthesis. Dosing of leucovorin depends on the individual protocol but is usually 12–15 mg/m^2 administered every 6 h starting 24–48 h after the MTX infusion and continuing until the plasma MTX concentration falls <0.05–0.1 μmol/L [1, 8, 9].

Renal clearance of MTX may be inhibited by the concomitant administration of the following medications, potentially leading to increased plasma levels of MTX and an increased risk of MTX associated toxicity [6, 8, 9]:

Nonsteroidal anti-inflammatory drugs (NSAIDs), e.g., ibuprofen, naproxen
Proton pump inhibitors, e.g., omeprazole, pantoprazole
Penicillins, e.g., amoxicillin, piperacillin, ticarcillin
Salicylates, e.g., acetylsalicylic acid (ASA)
Sulfonamides, e.g., co-trimoxazole, sulfamethoxazole, sulfisoxazole
Probenecid

Glucarpidase (formerly known as carboxypeptidase-G2) can be used to treat patients at risk for methotrexate toxicity secondary to delayed elimination (i.e., patients with HDMTX-induced renal failure and extremely elevated MTX levels). It is a recombinant bacterial enzyme that hydrolyzes MTX to an inactive metabolite. It can rapidly lower serum MTX levels by >95% within 15 min of administration [8, 10]. The dose is 50 units/kg given intravenously over 5 min. A second dose may be given within 24–48 h for MTX levels >100 μmol/L. High-dose leucovorin (1,000 mg/m^2 IV every 6 h) should be given 2–4 h before or after administration of glucarpidase [8, 10]. Glucarpidase is an investigational agent in Canada and can be obtained via the Health Canada Special Access Programme [8].

Hypersensitivity Reactions Related to Chemotherapeutic Agents

Hypersensitivity reactions (HSRs) to chemotherapeutic agents are defined as unexpected reactions with signs and symptoms not consistent with known toxicities of these drugs [11]. These reactions may affect any organ system in the body, and their severity ranges from mild flushing to anaphylaxis [11, 12]. Most chemotherapy drugs have the potential to cause HSRs [13], but there are groups of agents that have a high risk of such reactions, including the asparaginases, taxanes, platinum compounds, and epipodophyllotoxins [11–14]. The overall incidence of HSRs to chemotherapy drugs is reported to be approximately 5% [13]; however, this incidence is expected to rise as use of these agents in clinical practice continues to increase.

The exact mechanisms of hypersensitivity to chemotherapy are not fully understood. It appears that most acute reactions are related to type I hypersensitivity [11, 12]. (Table 13.3 summarizes the categories of HSRs.) Multiple factors such as drug form, route and rate of administration, and previous drug exposure affect the possibility of an HSR [11]. Excipients (i.e., substances used as diluent or a vehicle for a drug) such as Cremophor® (registered), EL in paclitaxel, and teniposide solutions have also been implicated as a potential cause of HSRs [11, 13, 14] (Tables 13.3 and 13.4).

Table 13.3 Categories of hypersensitivity reactions (HSRs) [12, 13]

Type of HSR	Mechanism of action	Signs and symptoms
I	Immediate hypersensitivity; IgE-mediated	Urticaria, pruritus, fever, anaphylaxis, angioedema, bronchospasm, hypotension
II	Antibody-mediated; IgG- or IgM-mediated	Hemolysis is most common
III	Immune-complex mediated	Vasculitis, nephritis, arthritis
IV	Delayed or cell-mediated; T lymphocyte activation	Graft rejection, contact dermatitis, granuloma formation

Ig immunoglobulin

Table 13.4 Main characteristics of hypersensitivity reactions to chemotherapeutic agents [11, 14]

Chemotherapy agent	Incidence of HSRs (%)	Time of initial onset	Description of HSR
L-asparaginase	6–43% (after IV administration; <10% are serious)	Within 1st hour of administration/2 weeks after initiation	Urticaria, rash (most occur after two weeks), flushing, bronchospasm, hypotension
Carboplatin	27	Within minutes to days/mostly after 7th course	Urticaria, rash (mostly after cycles 6–8), bronchospasm, hypotension, edema
Cisplatin	5–20	Within minutes/between 4th and 8th courses	Rash, pruritus, fever, cough, bronchospasm, hypotension
Oxaliplatin	10–20	Within minutes to hours/ after 8th course	Urticaria, fever, bronchospasm, rash, hypotension, hemolysis, joint pain
Docetaxel	25–50	First minutes of infusion/during 1st or 2nd cycle	Urticaria, bronchospasm, dyspnea, heart rate fluctuations, angioedema
Paclitaxel	8–45	First minutes of infusion/during 1st or 2nd cycle	Urticaria, bronchospasm, hypotension (common with 1st or 2nd dose), flushing, chest pain
Epipodophyllotoxins	0.7–14	After repeated exposure	Hypotension, bronchospasm, dyspnea, rash

Prevention of HSRs to chemotherapy is the primary goal, and protocols to prevent or reduce the severity of these reactions have been developed. The likelihood of an HSR increases with repeated exposure to L-asparaginase, platinum compounds, and the epipodophyllotoxins [13]. Skin testing can be performed on patients with a history of drug allergies or exposure to these agents. There are some reports of successful skin testing with carboplatin, oxaliplatin, and L-asparaginase, but this is not a standard practice as it has not been validated.

No standard desensitization protocols exist for chemotherapeutic agents. Many of the published recommendations are based on case reports with variable success [13]. There are also no standard premedication regimens to prevent HSRs to chemotherapy drugs, although several regimens have been proposed. Medications commonly used include corticosteroids (e.g., dexamethasone or equivalent), histamine 1 antagonists (e.g., diphenhydramine), histamine 2 antagonists (e.g., ranitidine), and antipyretics (e.g., acetaminophen). For example, premedication with a corticosteroid and an antihistamine is standard practice prior to administration of paclitaxel or docetaxel and successfully reduces the incidence of HSRs to 2–4% [13, 14]. However, premedication has not proven successful in prevention of HSRs with platinum compounds or epipodophyllotoxins [11, 13].

Table 13.5 Management of hypersensitivity reactions to chemotherapeutic agents [15]

General management of moderate HSR (e.g., moderate rash, flushing, pruritus, mild dyspnea, chest discomfort, abdominal discomfort, lower back pain, mild hypotension)	• Stop infusion • Give diphenhydramine 1 mg/kg (max 50 mg) and/or hydrocortisone sodium succinate 5–10 mg/kg (max 100 mg) IV push • After symptom recovery, resume infusion at rate as per protocol (if no protocol, consider resuming at 25% of previous rate for 5 min, 50% for 5 min, 75% for 5 min, and then full rate if no further reaction)
General management of severe (potentially life-threatening) HSR (e.g., one or more of respiratory distress requiring treatment, angioedema, hypotension requiring treatment)	• Stop infusion and do not restart • Give diphenhydramine 1 mg/kg (max 50 mg) and/or hydrocortisone sodium succinate 5–10 mg/kg (max 100 mg) IV push • Oxygen, if needed, for dyspnea • Normal saline, if needed, for hypotension • Epinephrine or bronchodilators, if indicated • Initiate emergency response system appropriate for facility, if patient condition warrants

In patients with a history of HSR to *E. coli*-derived L-asparaginase, a common strategy is to switch to a different preparation such as *Erwinia*-derived L-asparaginase or a polyethylene glycol–modified preparation (i.e., PEG-asparaginase) [11, 14]. Crossover reactions can occur in up to 23% of patients [11]. In some studies, docetaxel has been tolerated by patients who have had reactions to paclitaxel [13], but other studies have reported 90% cross-reactivity [11, 12, 14]. The true incidence of cross sensitivity between cisplatin and carboplatin is not defined because of limited studies [11, 14]. Successful substitution of carboplatin with cisplatin has been variable in preventing HSRs. The epipodophyllotoxins have not been found to develop cross-reactivity; however, because they are used to treat different cancers, they have not been substituted for one another [13].

HSRs to chemotherapeutic agents still happen despite the use of appropriate prevention strategies. Therefore, it is important to recognize these reactions quickly. In the event of an HSR, the primary intervention should be to discontinue the infusion of the offending agent while maintaining patent vascular access [12]. The ABCs of resuscitation (airway, breathing, and circulation) are then followed based on the patient's symptoms. Other first-line therapies for patients with severe HSRs include oxygen, epinephrine, and intravenous fluids (Table 13.5).

Extravasation (Paravasat)	Definitions
Extravasation	The inadvertent leakage or escape of a drug or fluid from a vein during intravenous administration [16, 17].
Vesicant	Agent capable of causing blistering, tissue damage, and/or necrosis after leakage into a vein or surrounding tissue.
Irritant	Agent that may cause pain in the vein or surrounding tissue, an inflammatory response with or without erythema, sclerosis, and hyperpigmentation along the vein during administration.
Flare	Painless local reaction along the vein or near the injection site, characterized by red blotches or streaks along the vessel with or without pruritus or irritation; symptoms usually subside 30 min after infusion is stopped.
Non-DNA-binding vesicants	e.g., *Vincristine, vinblastine* cause rapid tissue damage similar to a burn; injury is localized and heals without additional tissue damage.
DNA-binding vesicants	e.g., *Anthracyclines (doxorubicin, daunorubicin, idarubicin, mitoxantrone), antitumor antibiotics, and some alkylating agents* become trapped in the tissues and cause skin blistering and ulcer formation over several weeks; damage continues as necrotic tissue releases the drug over weeks, eventually extending to underlying tendons, ligaments, nerves, and bone, causing severe pain and functional deficit.

Extravasation of chemotherapeutic agents can be a rare but serious complication of cancer treatment. Although it is believed to be underreported, extravasation is estimated to occur in 0.1–0.6% of peripheral intravenous infusions and in 0.3–4.7% of implanted venous access device (VAD) infusions [17, 18]. Most incidents of extravasation are preventable. If an extravasation does occur, early and aggressive intervention is essential to minimize the risk of serious damage (Tables 13.6–13.8 and Fig. 13.1).

Cytotoxic spills	Definitions
Cytotoxic agent	A pharmacologic compound that is detrimental or destructive to cells within the body.
Cytotoxic waste	Unused cytotoxic drugs, tubing, needles, or other items that have come into contact with cytotoxic agents [20].
Exposure	Any contact with cytotoxic agents that may carry some health risk. Four potential routes of exposure to chemotherapy agents are inhalation, ingestion, injection, and absorption (through skin and eyes).
PPE	Personal protective equipment: items such as gloves, gowns, respirators, goggles, face shields, and others that protect individual workers from hazardous physical or chemical exposures.
Small spills	A small cytotoxic spill is defined as an incident resulting in a chemotherapy spill of quantities less than or equaling 100 mL. Proper cleanup should be performed by staff members (usually nurses) with the appropriate knowledge, skills, and equipment.
Large spills	A large spill is defined as any incident resulting in a chemotherapy spill of quantities more than 100 mL. Management of large spills may need to be coordinated through an external spill response agency.

Table 13.6 Assessment of extravasation versus other reactions [16, 19]

Assessment parameter	Extravasation Immediate extravasation	Delayed extravasation	Spasm/irritation of the vein	Flare reaction
Pain	Severe pain or burning lasting for minutes or hours, which eventually subsides; usually occurs around needle site while drug is being given	48 h	Aching and tightness along the vein	Ranges from no pain to aching
Redness	Blotchy redness around needle site; not always present at time of extravasation	Hours to months	Full length of vein may be reddened or darkened	Immediate blotches or streaks along vein, usually subsides within 30 min with or without treatment
Ulceration	Develops insidiously (usually occurs 48–96 h later)	Hours to months	Not usually	Not usually
Swelling	Severe swelling; usually occurs immediately	48 h	Not likely	Not likely; wheals may appear along vein line
Blood return	Inability to obtain blood return	Good blood return during administra-tion	Usually	Usually
Other	Change in quality of infusion	Local tingling and sensory deficits	Possible resistance felt on injection	Urticaria

Adapted from Oncology Nursing Society (ONS) Cancer Chemotherapy Guidelines

Table 13.7 Categories of chemotherapy agents based on extravasation risk

Vesicant	Nonvesicant Irritant	None	
Amsacrine	Bortezimib	Aldesleukin (IL-2)	Interferon
Busulfan	Cisplatin	Asparaginase	Leucovorin
Carmustine	Dacarbazine	Azacytidine	Leuprolide
Dactinomycin	Docetaxel	BCG	Methotrexate
Daunorubicin	Etoposide	Bevacizumab	Rituximab
Doxorubicin	Fluorouracil	Bleomycin	Thiotepa
Epirubicin	Ifosfamide	Carboplatin	Topotecan
Idarubicin	Irinotecan	Cladribine	Trastuzumab
Mechlorethamine	Mitoxantrone	Clofarabine	
Melphalan	Oxaliplatin	Cyclophosphamide	
Mitomycin	Paclitaxel	Cytarabine	
Vinblastine	Temozolomide	Dexrazoxane	
Vincristine	Teniposide	Fludarabine	
Vinorelbine		Gemcitabine	

Table 13.8 Medication-specific management of extravasation [16, 18, 19]

Chemotherapy agent	Local care	Antidote recommended	Comments
Cisplatin	Cold compress	Sodium thiosulfate To prepare 4.1% solution, mix 1.6 mL of 25% sodium thiosulfate with 8.4 mL of sterile water for injection or 0.9% NaCl	Elevate site of extravasation Antidote only indicated for large-volume (> 20 mL) extravasations of a concentrated solution (>0.4 mg/mL) Administer through existing IV line
Daunorubicin Doxorubicin Idarubicin Mitoxantrone	Cold compress	Dimethylsulfoxide (DMSO) 50% Apply 4 drops/10 cm² skin surface to site 3–4 times/day for 7–14 days. Allow to air-dry. Do not cover	Elevate site of extravasation Do not apply heat; it may worsen injury Protect from heat and sunlight Corticosteroids worsen toxicity Avoid direct contact with DMSO (double gloves and metal forceps)
Mitomycin-C	None	Dimethylsulfoxide (DMSO) 50% Apply 4 drops/10 cm² skin surface to site 3–4 times/day for 7–14 days. Allow to air-dry. Do not cover	Elevate site of extravasation Do not apply heat; it may worsen injury Protect from heat and sunlight Avoid direct contact with DMSO (double gloves and metal forceps)
Epipodophyllotoxins (etoposide, teniposide)	Warm compress	Hyaluronidase Reconstitute to 150 units/mL Prepare 5-mL × 0.2-mL injections and inject around site Not for IV administration	Elevate site of extravasation Hyaluronidase only for large-volume extravasations of concentrated solutions Immediate onset of action with a 24–48-h duration
Mechlorethamine	None	Sodium thiosulfate To prepare 4.1% solution, mix 1.6 mL of 25% sodium thiosulfate with 8.4 mL of sterile water for injection or 0.9% NaCl	Elevate site of extravasation Timely administration is crucial Administer through existing IV line

(continued)

Table 13.8 (continued)

Chemotherapy agent	Local care	Antidote recommended	Comments
Paclitaxel	Cold compress (ice pack for 15–20 min at least four times/ day × 24 h)	Hyaluronidase Reconstitute to 150 units/ mL Prepare 5-mL × 0.2-mL injections and inject around site Not for IV administration	Elevate site of extravasation Immediate onset of action with a 24–48-h duration
Vinblastine Vincristine Vinorelbine	Warm compress	Hyaluronidase Reconstitute to 150 units/ mL Prepare 5-mL × 0.2-mL injections and inject around site Not for IV administration	Elevate site of extravasation Corticosteroids and topical cooling worsen toxicity Immediate onset of action with a 24–48-h duration
Carmustine Dactinomycin Dacarbazine Docetaxel Melphalan	Cold compress	None	Elevate site of extravasation Protect from heat and sunlight
Oxaliplatin	None	None	Elevate site of extravasation DO NOT APPLY COLD. Cold can precipitate acute neurotoxicity Early administration of corticosteroids may be beneficial to decrease inflammation

Cytotoxic drug spills should be managed according to established, written policies and procedures for each workplace. Cytotoxic spill kits must be available in all areas where cytotoxic drugs are prepared, dispensed, administered, received, stored, and disposed. Spills involving these agents should be cleaned by staff members with the appropriate knowledge, skills, and equipment. The size of the spill might determine who is authorized to conduct the cleanup and decontamination and how the cleanup is managed (Tables 13.9 and 13.10).

Fig. 13.1 Management algorithm for suspected extravasation of chemotherapy

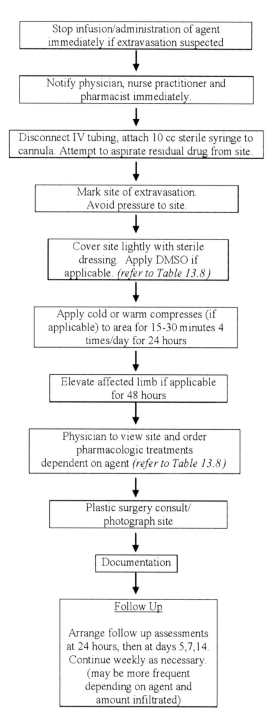

Table 13.9 Equipment/supplies recommended for cytotoxic spill cleanup [21, 22, 23]

Personal protective equipment (PPE)		Other supplies	
Hands	Chemotherapy-approved powder-free gloves along with snug fitting cuffs, made of latex or nitrile NIOSH standards recommend double gloving, with the outer glove extending over the cuff of the gown	Chemotherapy Drug Spill Kit	Should include 2-pair gloves, gown, shoe coverings
Body	Disposable gowns made of polyethylene-coated polypropylene (nonlinting and nonabsorbent). Gowns should have closed fronts, long sleeves, and elastic or knit-closed cuffs	Cleaning supplies	Hospital detergent solution, disposable absorbent pads, bucket, and mop
Eye/face	Face shield or goggles. Goggles only protect eyes, while face shield protects eyes, nose, and mouth. Wear in addition to corrective eyewear	Sharps	Reusable or disposable cytotoxic sharps container
Respiratory	A hospital approved, individually fit tested N95 respirator	Waste container and labels	Dispose all spill cleanup materials in a hazardous chemical waste container
	A surgical mask does not offer respiratory protection		Label all waste with cytotoxic stickers
Feet	Disposable shoe coverings	Material safety data sheet (MSDS)	Contains summaries provided by the manufacturer to describe properties and hazards of specific chemicals and ways workers can protect themselves from exposure to these chemicals

NIOSH National Institute for Occupational Safety and Health

Table 13.10 Recommended cytotoxic spill cleanup procedures [20, 21]

A. Preparation	1. Collect equipment and supplies
	2. Follow Spill Kit instructions
	3. Restrict access to spill area and post appropriate signs
	4. Put on PPE
B. Contain spill	Liquid spills – lay absorbent pads over spill to absorb the liquid and turn it into a gel
	Solid spills – gently cover and remove powder spills with damp absorbent pads; wipe solids with wet absorbent pads
	Sharps – use a scoop to place broken glass into a cytotoxic sharps container
C. Clean area	Initial cleanup: Clean spill area and nondisposable items three times with disinfectant solution and absorbent pads
	Final cleanup: Rinse area twice with clean water
D. Disposal	Place contaminated absorbent pads and all PPE in appropriate hazardous waste container or bag. Label with cytotoxic sticker
	Any disposable items that have come in contact with cytotoxic agent (e.g., linens) should be disposed of in hazardous waste container
E. Documentation (e.g., Safety Occurrence Report)	• Agent and volume spilled
	• Immediate and basic causes of spill
	• Spill management procedures followed
	• Personnel, patient, and others exposed to the spill
	• Corrective actions implemented to prevent a similar occurrence in future

References

1. Balis FM, Holcenberg JS, Blaney SM. General Principles of Chemotherapy. In: Pizzo PA, Poplack DG, eds. Principles and Practice of Pediatric Oncology. 4th ed. Philadelphia, Pa: Lippincott Williams & Wilkins; 2002:237–308.

2. Moore MJ, Goldenberg GJ. Antineoplastic Drugs. In: Kalant H, Roschlau WHE, eds. Principles of Medical Pharmacology.6th ed. New York, NY: Oxford University Press; 1998:759–774.

3. What are the different types of chemotherapy drugs.http://www.cancer.org/Treatment/TreatmentsandSideEffects/TreatmentTypes/Chemotherapy/index. Accessed November 29, 2010.

4. Ivy SP, Lugo TG, Bernstein ML, Smith MA. Evolving Molecular and Targeted Therapies. In: Pizzo PA, Poplack DG, eds. Principles and Practice of Pediatric Oncology.4th ed. Philadelphia, Pa: Lippincott Williams & Wilkins; 2002:309–349.

5. Biological Therapy Agents.http://training.seer.cancer.gov/treatment/biotherapy/agents.html. Accessed November 29, 2010.

6. Beorlegui B, Aldaz A, Ortega A, et al.Potential interaction between methotrexate and omeprazole. The Annals of Pharmacotherapy.2000;34:1024–1027.

7. Blum R, Seymour JF, Toner G. Significant impairment of high-dose methotrexate clearance following vancomycin administration in the absence of overt renal impairment. Annals of Oncology.2002;13:327–330.

8. BC Cancer Agency Cancer Drug Manual.http://www.bccancer.bc.ca/HPI/DrugDatabase/DrugIndexPro/Methotrexate.htm.Accessed November 29, 2010.

9. Commercial Agents Monographs for the Children's Oncology Group.https://member.children-soncologygroup.org/_files/disc/Pharmacy/CommercialAgentsMonographsV3.pdf.Accessed November 29, 2010.

10. Widemann BC, Balis FM, Murphy RF, et al.Carboxypeptidase-G2, thymidine, and leucovorin rescue in cancer patients with methotrexate-induced renal dysfunction. Journal of Clinical Oncology.1997;15(5):2125–2134.

11. Syrigou E, Triantafyllou O, Makrilia N, et al.Acute hypersensitivity reactions to chemotherapy agents: an overview. Inflammation & Allergy – Drug Targets.2010;9:206–213.

12. Zanotti KM, Markman M. Prevention and management of antineoplastic-induced hypersensitivity reactions. Drug Safety.2001;24(10):767–779.

13. Gobel BH. Chemotherapy-induced hypersensitivity reactions. Oncology Nursing Forum.2005;32(5):1027–1034.

14. Lee C, Gianos M, Klaustermeyer WB. Diagnosis and management of hypersensitivity reactions related to common cancer chemotherapy agents. Ann Allergy Asthma Immunol.2009;102:179–187.

15. BCCA protocol summary for management of hypersensitivity reactions to chemotherapeutic agents. In: de Lemos M, Badry N, ed.B.C. Cancer Agency Cancer Drug Manual. 2nd ed. Vancouver, BC:B.C. Cancer Agency, Division of Pharmacy, 2010.

16. ONC – Cytotoxic Agents – Prevention and management of vesicant extravasation.http://policy.hhsc.ca/default.aspx?page = 11&class27.IdType = policy&class27.Id = 48828.Accessed December 11, 2010.

17. Guideline for the prevention and management of chemotherapy extravasation in children and young people receiving cancer treatment.http://www.yorkshire-cancer-net.org.uk/html/down-loads/ycn_hyccn_cyp_haematology_oncology_guidelinesextravastaion_sept2008.pdf. Accessed December 11, 2010.

18. Extravasation guidelines.https://members.childrensoncologygroup.org/_files/disc/Nursing/extravasationguidelines.pdf.Accessed December 15, 2010.

19. Extravasation of chemotherapy, prevention and management of. In: de Lemos M, Badry N, ed.B.C. Cancer Agency Cancer Drug Manual. 2nd ed. Vancouver, BC: B.C. Cancer Agency, Division of Pharmacy, 2010.

20. HSW – Spill Response Protocol.http://policy.hhsc.ca/default.aspx?page = 11&class27. Id = 63013.Accessed December 15, 2010.

21. Cytotoxic Agents: Safe handling policy – segregation, preparation, transportation and waste disposal.http://policy.hhsc.ca/default.aspx?page = 11&class27.IdType = policy&class27. ID = 51739.Accessed December 15, 2010.

22. The University of Texas M.D. Anderson Cancer Center.PPE and management of chemotherapy spills policy, UTMDACC institutional policy # ADM0171, 1–12.

23. Ettinger AG, Bond DM, Sievers TD. Chemotherapy. In: Baggott CR, Kelly KP, Fochtman D, Foley GV, eds. Nursing Care of Children and Adolescents with Cancer.3rd ed. Philadelphia, Pa: W.B. Wanders Company; 2002:133–176.

Chapter 14
Supportive Care

Paula MacDonald

Keywords 5-HT$_3$ receptor • Anticipatory emesis • *Candida* sp. • Electrolyte replacement • Granulocyte colony-stimulating factor (G-CSF) • Medullary bone pain • Myelosuppression • Nausea • Oral magnesium supplementation • Pneumocystis prophylaxis • Prolonged neutropenia • Splenomegaly • Thrombocytopenia • Trimethoprim-sulfamethoxazole • Vomiting

Introduction

The treatment of cancer is commonly associated with pain, nausea, and other distressing symptoms. Therefore, a primary goal in the medical management of pediatric cancer patients is symptom management through supportive care. Aggressive supportive care can improve outcomes for children with cancer, especially in high-risk patients. For example, nausea and vomiting are considered by many patients to be among the most debilitating side effects of chemotherapy and radiation. The impact of inadequately controlled nausea and vomiting on patients' quality of life is substantial, and administration of prophylactic antiemetics has become a standard of supportive care in children receiving treatment for cancer. The use of prophylaxis against *Pneumocystis jirovecii* (formerly *carinii*) pneumonia (PCP) has also become a routine part of management of many childhood cancers. Other supportive measures commonly required in the care of pediatric oncology patients include fungal prophylaxis, electrolyte supplementation, administration of prophylactic granulocyte colony-stimulating factor (G-CSF), and therapeutic amenorrhea.

P. MacDonald (✉)
Division of Hematology/Oncology, McMaster Children's Hospital,
1200 Main Street West, Hamilton, ON, Canada L8N 3Z5
e-mail: macdonap@hhsc.ca

K. Scheinemann and A.E. Boyce (eds.), *Emergencies in Pediatric Oncology*, 121
DOI 10.1007/978-1-4614-1174-1_14, © Springer Science+Business Media, LLC 2012

Antiemetics	Definitions
Nausea:	Subjective symptom described as recognition or feeling of the imminent need to vomit [1, 2].
Vomiting:	The forceful expulsion of gastric contents as a consequence of complex reflex actions initiated by the vomiting center in the medulla [1].
Retching:	The attempt at vomiting, without expulsion of gastric contents [1].

Nausea and vomiting are two of the most distressing side effects experienced by cancer patients despite major advances that have led to improved pharmacological options for control of these symptoms. Nausea often occurs with vomiting; however, either can occur independently. Without effective prophylaxis, these symptoms can lead to severe dehydration, electrolyte imbalances, and emotional or psychological distress. Chemotherapy and radiation are well-known causes of nausea and vomiting; however, cancer patients may also experience these symptoms secondary to metastatic disease, increased intracranial pressure, metabolic disturbances, delayed gastric emptying, gastrointestinal obstruction, anesthetic agents, and opioids [1, 2]. Psychological factors (i.e., anxiety and patient's prior experiences with nausea and vomiting) can also contribute to chemotherapy-induced nausea and vomiting (CINV).

Pathophysiology of Nausea and Vomiting

Vomiting occurs when central or peripheral neurologic pathways stimulate the vomiting center located in the brainstem [1]. Chemotherapeutic agents induce vomiting by stimulating the vomiting center directly or by stimulation of the chemotherapy trigger zone (CTZ) located in the floor of the fourth ventricle in the vicinity of the area postrema [2]. Chemotherapy causes the release of emetic neurotransmitters that stimulate the CTZ which in turn activates the vomiting center to produce nausea and vomiting [1, 2]. Neurotransmitters that stimulate the CTZ include serotonin (5-HT), dopamine (D_2), histamine (H_1), and acetylcholine (ACh) [3]. Enterochromaffin cells in the intestinal mucosa are rich in 5-HT and D_2 receptors, and damage induced by chemotherapy, radiation, or bowel distension can result in a massive release of (5-HT) [3].

Chemotherapy-induced nausea and vomiting can be acute, delayed, or anticipatory. *Acute* symptoms occur during the first 24 h after chemotherapy administration and tend to be responsive to drug therapy. *Delayed* nausea and vomiting occur more than 24 h after treatment and can persist for several days. It is less common in children than in adults [3] and is not very responsive to drug therapy. Most patients experience delayed symptoms after receiving cisplatin. *Anticipatory* emesis occurs before chemotherapy is given and is difficult to treat because it is a conditioned response that may be related to anxiety. More than half of pediatric cancer patients experience anticipatory symptoms [2]. Conditioned responses are more likely if nausea and vomiting with early chemotherapy cycles is not well controlled. Antiemetics do not effectively control anticipatory symptoms once they have developed.

Therefore, effective prevention of acute nausea and vomiting can reduce the risk of delayed or anticipatory symptoms [2, 3].

The incidence and severity of CINV are affected by both patient- and treatment-related factors. A higher risk is associated with female gender, age greater than 3 years, anxiety, history of motion sickness, and poor control with previous chemotherapy [3]. Treatment-related risk factors include the emetogenicity, schedule, dose, route, and rate of drug administration. The most important factor is the intrinsic emetogenicity of the chemotherapy agent. Table 14.1 summarizes the emetogenic potential of commonly used chemotherapeutic agents. Antiemetics are most effective when given prophylactically; therefore, routine use of antiemetics is recommended for pediatric patients receiving emetogenic chemotherapy and radiation to the brain and abdomen/pelvis [4]. When these chemotherapy agents are used in combination, antiemetic prophylaxis should be based on the most emetic component of the regimen. Antiemetic regimens should also be individualized based on patient tolerance.

The following factors should be considered when selecting an antiemetic regimen:

1. Emetogenic potential of chemotherapeutic agents and/or radiation
2. Patient's tolerance of previous chemotherapy
3. Expected onset and duration of nausea and vomiting
4. Presence of anticipatory nausea and vomiting
5. Concomitant medications or medical conditions that increase risk of symptoms
6. History of allergy or adverse reaction to antiemetic agents

The primary goal of antiemetic therapy is complete prevention of treatment-related nausea and vomiting. The combination of a 5-HT_3 receptor antagonist with dexamethasone is the standard of care for prevention of acute CINV induced by moderate to highly emetogenic chemotherapy in children. Lorazepam and diphenhydramine are useful adjuncts to the antiemetic regimen but are not recommended as single agents. Metoclopramide, prochlorperazine, and cannabinoids should be reserved for patients intolerant of or refractory to first-line antiemetics. All antiemetics, with the exception of aprepitant, should be administered on a routine schedule ("round-the-clock"), not as needed ("prn"), for at least 24 h after chemotherapy [10].

Novel or emerging agents, including metopimazine, olanzapine, and gabapentin, may have a future role to play in emetic control. However, there is insufficient published pediatric experience with these agents for the prevention of CINV, and they are not currently considered for routine use [7] (Table 14.2).

Pneumocystis Prophylaxis

Pneumocystis jirovecii (formerly *carinii*) pneumonia (PCP) is a serious complication in pediatric oncology patients. Children and adolescents with cancer are at an increased risk for developing this opportunistic infection due to immunosuppression

Table 14.1 Emetogenicity of chemotherapeutic agents and radiation therapy [3–6]

Very high risk (>90% frequency)	High risk (60–90% frequency)	Moderate risk (30–60% frequency)	Moderate to low (10–30% frequency)	Low risk (<10% frequency)
Carmustine ($\geq$200 mg/m^2)	Carboplatin	Cyclophosphamide ($\leq$ 750 mg/m^2)	Bortezomib	Asparaginase
Cisplatin ($\geq$50 mg/m^2)	Carmustine (<200 mg/m^2)	Dactinomycin ($\leq$ 1.5 mg/m^2)	Cytarabine (<1 g/m^2)	Bleomycin
Cyclophosphamide (>1.500 mg/m^2)	Cisplatin (<50 mg/m^2)	Doxorubicin (20–60 mg/m^2)	Daunorubicin (<45 mg/m^2)	Busulfan (oral)
Dacarbazine ($\geq$500 mg/m^2)	Clofarabine	Idarubicin	Docetaxel	Cladribine
Ifosfamide ($\geq$1.500 mg/m^2)	Cyclophosphamide (>750 & $\leq$ 1.500 mg/m^2)	Ifosfamide (<1.500 mg/m^2)	Doxorubicin (<20 mg/m^2)	Cyclophosphamide (oral)
Lomustine (>60 mg/m^2)	Cytarabine ($\geq$1 g/m^2)	Methotrexate (250–1,000 mg/m^2)	Etoposide	Cytarabine (<100 mg/m^2)
Mechlorethamine	Dactinomycin (>1.5 mg/m^2)		Fluorouracil ($\leq$ 1 g/m^2)	Dexrazoxane
	Dacarbazine (<500 mg/m^2)		Gemcitabine	Fludarabine
	Daunorubicin ($\geq$45 mg/m^2)		Methotrexate (>50 & < 250 mg/m^2)	Gefitinib
	Doxorubicin (>60 mg/m^2)		Mitomycin (<8 mg/m^2)	Hydroxyurea
	Irinotecan		Mitoxantrone	Imatinib
	Lomustine ($\leq$ 60 mg/m^2)		Nelarabine	Isotretinoin
	Methotrexate (>1 g/m^2)		Paclitaxel	Methotrexate (<50 mg/m^2)
	Mitomycin ($\geq$8 mg/m^2)		Teniposide	Melphalan
	Oxaliplatin (>75 mg/m^2)		Thiotepa	Mercaptopurine
	Procarbazine		Topotecan	Rituximab
	Total body irradiation (TBI)		Triple intrathecal chemotherapy	Sorafenib
			Abdominal/pelvic or craniospinal irradiation	Temozolamide
				Thioguanine
				Trastuzumab
				Vinblastine
				Vincristine
				Vinorelbine
				Head/neck/cranial/extremities irradiation

Table 14.2 Antiemetic medications [1–10]

Antiemetic agent	Efficacy/indications	Route, frequency, and dose	Adverse effects/limitations to Use
Serotonin (5-HT$_3$) receptor antagonists	Most effective antiemetics for acute CINV; well-established efficacy for radiation-induced emesis; reduced efficacy for delayed nausea and vomiting	Oral and intravenous dosing (Ondansetron also available as oral dissolving tablet (ODT))	Low incidence of side effects; generally well tolerated
Ondansetron		Ondansetron 0.15 mg/kg every 8 h (maximum of 8 mg/dose) or 0.45 mg/kg (maximum of 32 mg IV or 24 mg PO) once daily	Most common: headache, constipation, drowsiness
Granisetron			Transient elevated liver enzymes (asymptomatic)
Dolasetron (available in Canada)	Efficacy enhanced by combination with steroids for prevention of acute CINV		Tachycardia, bradycardia, hypotension reported with ondansetron
Tropisetron and palonosetron are not on market in Canada (further pediatric research required)	Most pediatric experience with ondansetron and granisetron	Granisetron 10–20 mcg/kg every 12 h (maximum of 1 mg/dose) or 20–40 mcg/kg (maximum of 2 mg) once daily	Electrocardiographic (ECG) abnormalities, although do not appear to be of clinical significance
	For prevention of acute emesis, equivalent doses have equivalent safety and efficacy; may be used interchangeably	Dolasetron 1.8 mg/kg (maximum of 100 mg/dose) as a single dose pre-chemo	Dolasetron IV contraindicated secondary to risk of abnormal heart rhythm (torsade de pointes)[6]
		Administer 30 min prior to chemo if IV and 1 h prior if oral	
		Emerging data suggest that oral route is as efficacious as IV route	
Corticosteroids	Mechanism unknown	Oral and intravenous dosing	Routine use discouraged in leukemia, lymphoma, brain tumor patients (may reduce delivery of chemotherapy to brain tumors by repairing the blood–brain barrier)
Dexamethasone	Synergistic activity with 5-HT$_3$ antagonists and metoclopramide (20% increase in efficacy for acute CINV)[7]	No clear dose guidelines for children Dexamethasone: Low dose: 2.5–3 mg/m^2 (maximum of 4 mg/dose) every 12 h	
Methylprednisolone	More effective for delayed symptoms than 5-HT$_3$ antagonists	High dose: 4.5–8 mg/m^{2}dose (maximum of 8 mg/dose) every 8–12 h	Most common: insomnia, heartburn and agitation; also hyperglycemia. increased appetite, mood and behavioral disturbances reported
	Also effective for radiation-induced emesis	May substitute with methylprednisolone (ratio 5:1 with dexamethasone)	

(continued)

Table 14.2 (continued)

Antiemetic agent	Efficacy/indications	Route, frequency, and dose	Adverse effects/limitations to Use
Dopamine Antagonist Metoclopramide	Efficacy with moderately emetogenic regimens	Oral and intravenous dosing 1–2 mg/kg/dose every 2–4 h if needed (prn)	Risk of acute dystonic reactions in children and extrapyramidal symptoms (administer with diphenhydramine)
	Efficacy in delayed nausea and vomiting	Delayed CINV: 0.1–0.2 mg/kg/dose every 6 h	Sedation, dry mouth, diarrhea, hypotension
	Inferior to 5-HT$_3$ antagonists for radiation-induced emesis		
Antiemetic agent	Efficacy/indications	Route, frequency, and dose	Adverse effects/limitations to Use
Phenothiazines Prochlorperazine Promethazine	Most effective against mild to moderately emetogenic treatments	Oral and intravenous dosing Prochlorperazine 0.1 mg/kg every 6 h (maximum of 10 mg/dose)	Use limited by side effects Extrapyramidal symptoms, dystonic reactions in children (administer with diphenhydramine)
	Used for breakthrough nausea and vomiting	Promethazine 0.25–1 mg/kg every 4–6 h (maximum of 25/dose)	High incidence of orthostatic hypotension, sedation, restlessness
Benzodiazepines Lorazepam	Adjuncts to conventional antiemetics for breakthrough and refractory nausea and vomiting	Oral and intravenous dosing 0.025–0.05 mg/kg (maximum of 2 mg/ dose) every 6–12 h as needed (prn)	Sedation, drowsiness, motor incoordination, amnesia, respiratory depression
	Effective for anticipatory nausea, vomiting		Caution with additive sedation and respiratory depression with other antiemetics and narcotics
Antihistamines Dimenhydrinate Diphenhydramine	Mild antiemetic properties	Oral and intravenous dosing 1 mg/kg/dose every 4–6 h as needed (prn) (maximum of 50 mg/dose)	Drowsiness, sedation, dry mouth, hypotension, palpitations, tachycardia, urinary retention
	Used in combination with other antiemetics to potentiate effectiveness in refractory mild to moderate nausea		May increase CNS depression
	Used with dopamine antagonists to prevent extrapyramidal reactions		

Cannabinoids Nabilone	Derivatives of marijuana Exact mechanism unknown; weak to modest antiemetic efficacy; superior to metoclopramide, prochlorperazine, and domperidone Effective in management of anticipatory nausea and vomiting Particularly effective in adolescents and young adults refractory to standard antiemetic therapy	Oral only Twice daily dosing <12 years of age: <18 kg – 0.5 mg >18 kg – 1 mg ≥12 year of age: 1–2 mg/dose Start the night before chemotherapy	Use limited by adverse effect profile Drowsiness, dysphoria, dizziness, mood alteration, hypotension, tachycardia
Neurokinin-1 (NK-1) receptor antagonist Aprepitant	Effective in preventing cisplatin-induced nausea and vomiting in conjunction with 5-HT$_3$ antagonist and steroid; increased control of acute nausea by 10–15% and delayed nausea by 20–30% Insufficient data on pharmacokinetics, efficacy, and safety in young children	Oral only In patients >40 kg and ≥12 years, 125 mg x 1 on day of most highly emetogenic chemotherapy, then 80 mg daily on subsequent 2 days Optimal effective pediatric dose in young children unknown	Potentially significant drug interactions. Do not give the following drugs concurrently or for 2 weeks after aprepitant: Etoposide, ifosfamide, imatinib, irinotecan, vincristine, vinblastine, vinorelbine, phenytoin, carbamazepine, paclitaxel, phenobarbital, warfarin, benzodiazepines, clarithromycin, rifampin, oral contraceptives *Reduce corticosteroids by 25% if IV or 50% if oral while on aprepitant Asthenia/fatigue, dizziness, hiccups, heartburn, diarrhea, transient increase in LFTs reported

*IV intravenous

secondary to their underlying disease and exposure to corticosteroids or high-intensity chemotherapy regimens. There is still a high mortality rate (24%) associated with PCP despite early diagnosis and appropriate treatment with high-dose trimethoprim-sulfamethoxazole (TMP-SMX) [11]. Therefore, it is crucial that prophylaxis against PCP should begin at the initiation of chemotherapy and continue for at least three months following discontinuation of immunosuppressive therapy [4]. TMP-SMX is the best choice for PCP prophylaxis because of its safety profile, proven efficacy in children with cancer, and relative ease of administration. For patients 1–2 months of age, those allergic to TMP-SMX, with G-6PD deficiency, or experiencing excessive myelosuppression with TMP-SMX, alternative prophylaxis with dapsone, aerosolized or intravenous pentamidine, or atovaquone may be considered. No alternative regimen is as effective as TMP-SMX (Table 14.3).

Antifungal Prophylaxis in Pediatric Oncology Patients

Invasive fungal infections are a major cause of infection-related morbidity and mortality in pediatric oncology patients. Risk of these infections is related to intensity of chemotherapy regimens and duration of neutropenia [18, 19]. Other established risk factors for fungal infections in this patient population include the presence of indwelling central venous access devices, use of broad-spectrum antibiotics, corticosteroids, fungal colonization, and chemotherapy-induced mucositis [19, 20]. Patients with acute myeloid leukemia (AML) are at particularly high risk of invasive fungal infections. The predominant fungal pathogens in North America and Europe are *Candida* and *Aspergillus* species [2, 18]. Systemic antifungal prophylaxis has been shown to reduce morbidity and fungal-related mortality in severely neutropenic chemotherapy patients. Evidence for benefit is greatest for those with a >15% rate of systemic fungal infection, prolonged neutropenia, and stem cell transplant (SCT) recipients [4].

Most prophylactic regimens are aimed at reducing invasive infections caused by *Candida* sp. Topical agents (i.e., nystatin) have been widely used for prevention of mucosal candidiasis but effectiveness in preventing invasive fungal infections is controversial. Therefore, nystatin and clotrimazole troches are not recommended for fungal prophylaxis in high-risk patients [4]. Fluconazole, a systemically active antifungal triazole, is the most frequently studied prophylactic drug and is significantly better than nystatin at preventing invasive fungal infection. Table 14.4 summarizes antifungal agents for prophylaxis. The choice of prophylactic regimen should be made in consultation with specific institutional infection profiles and infectious disease guidelines.

There is concern that long-term use of prophylaxis may induce resistance to antifungal drugs and shift the colonization pattern of fungal organisms toward more resistant fungi. Susceptible fungi may be eradicated, permitting overgrowth of more resistant species (i.e., *Candida glabrata, Candida krusei, Candida parapsilosis, Aspergillus*). This has not yet been observed in clinical practice [19].

Table 14.3 Medications for PCP prophylaxis in pediatric oncology patients [11–17]

Medication	Efficacy	Dosing for PCP prophylaxis	Side effects/precautions
Trimethoprim-sulfamethoxazole (cotrimoxazole, TMP-SMX)	Drug of choice (first-line agent) Highly effective in preventing PCP 91–100% reported reduction in occurrence of PCP <10% breakthrough infection rate with compliant patients	2.5 mg TMP component/kg/dose orally twice a day given 3 days per week (75 mg TMP component/m^2/dose) Maximum of 160 mg of TMP component per dose	Bone marrow suppression (neutropenia, thrombocytopenia) Mild cutaneous rash, pruritus, fever Gastrointestinal upset (nausea, vomiting, diarrhea) Hyperkalemia ↑ Photosensitivity Transaminase elevation Stevens–Johnson syndrome (rare)
Dapsone	Recommended second-line agent for patients unable to tolerate TMP-SMX 10–15% breakthrough rate Preferred in patients < 2 months old because of liver prematurity	2 mg/kg/day orally (or 5–10 mg/kg/week divided 3 days per week) Maximum of 100 mg/day May also be given as 4 mg/kg/day once weekly (maximum of 200 mg/week)	Rash, fever Hepatic dysfunction Gastrointestinal upset Methemoglobinemia (cyanosis, headaches, dizziness, fatigue, weakness) Hemolytic anemia (dose-related hemolysis) Contraindicated in patients with G6PD deficiency
Aerosolized (inhaled) pentamidine	Breakthrough PCP rates 5–25% One study reported 2.7% breakthrough rate Does not prevent extrapulmonary infection	≥5 years: 300 mg monthly <5 years: 8 mg/kg monthly (maximum 300 mg per dose)	Bronchospasm, cough, wheezing Limited to children old enough to use the nebulizer
Intravenous pentamidine	Limited evaluation in pediatric oncology patients Reported breakthrough PCP rate of 1.3–2%	4 mg/kg/dose IV every 2 to 4 weeks Administered over 1–2 h; RN monitoring required during infusion for adverse effects	Hypoglycemia and hypotension during rapid infusion Hypercalcemia, hyper-kalemia, hypoglycemia Hypotension Nephrotoxicity Pancreatitis Dysrhythmias Transaminase elevations
Atovaquone	Limited evaluation in pediatric oncology patients Efficacy comparable to dapsone or aerosolized pentamidine	1–3 months: 30 mg/kg/day 4–24 months: 45 mg/kg/day >24 months: 30 mg/kg/day As a single daily dose (maximum of 1,500 mg/dose) Give with food to ensure adequate absorption	Favorable side effect profile (less toxic than dapsone) Most common side effect is mild upper gastrointestinal symptoms Fever, rash, transaminase elevation reported

Table 14.4 Antifungal agents for prophylaxis [2, 4, 18–21]

Agent	Spectrum	Efficacy	Prophylactic dosing	Side effects/precautions/drug interactions
Fluconazole	• Active against *Candida* • Active against dimorphic fungi (e.g., histoplasmosis, coccidioidomycosis) and *C. neoformans* Inactive against molds (e.g., *Aspergillus*, Zygomycetes)	Effectively controls colonization; reduces mucosal infections and invasive disease; reduces all-cause mortality Recommended first-line agent in pediatrics[4]	5 mg/kg/day orally or intravenously (maximum of 400 mg/day)	Variable resistance with *C. glabrata*; *C. Krusei* always resistant Side effects include nausea, vomiting, headache, dizziness, pruritus and rash, increased liver enzymes, and increased BUN and creatinine Drug–drug interactions common (inhibitor of CYP P450 isoenzymes)
Itraconazole	• Active against *Candida* and *Aspergillus* sp. • Active against dimorphic fungi and *C. neoformans* Poor activity vs. Zygomycetes	Reduced invasive fungal infections and *Candida* infections better than fluconazole Comparable effect on all-cause mortality vs. fluconazole	In children >5 years of age 2.5 mg/kg twice a day orally (maximum of 200 mg/dose)	Adverse gastrointestinal effects limit use Contraindicated in patients with significant cardiac systolic dysfunction Drug–drug interactions common (inhibitor of CYP P450 isoenzymes) Serum concentration monitoring recommended
Voriconazole	• Active against *Candida* and *Aspergillus* sp. • Active against dimorphic fungi and *C. neoformans* Poor activity vs. Zygomycetes	No studies for prophylaxis Standard of care as primary therapy for invasive aspergillosis	<20 kg: 50 mg IV/per os twice daily ≥20 kg: 100 mg IV/per os twice daily	Caution with IV form in patients with significant renal dysfunction; may worsen azotemia Serious hepatic reactions (i.e., hepatitis, cholestasis) – monitor transaminases and bilirubin closely Drug–drug interactions common (inhibitor of CYP P450 isoenzymes)

Drug	Activity	Prophylactic efficacy	Dosing	Comments
Posaconazole	• Active against *Candida*, *Aspergillus* sp. and some Zygomycetes sp. • Active against dimorphic fungi and *C. neoformans*	Effective prophylaxis in neutropenic MDS, AML, and HSCT recipients with significant GVHD (adult) but efficacy in pediatrics not established	200 mg three times daily orally (≥13 years of age)	No pediatric dosing information available for prophylaxis (safety not established) Should be administered with a full meal or liquid nutritional supplement
Amphotericin B formulations[a]	Broad spectrum of antifungal activity versus *Candida*, *Aspergillus* sp., Zygomycetes, rarer molds, *C. neoformans*, and dimorphic fungi	Insufficient data for prophylactic efficacy in pediatrics	No standardized pediatric dosing information for prophylaxis IV administration required	Substantial infusional and renal toxicity, although this is reduced with lipid formulations Hypokalemia common Requires frequent monitoring of renal function, electrolytes and hepatic function Lipid formulations very expensive
Caspofungin Micafungin Anidulafungin (echinocandins)	Active against *Candida* and *Aspergillus* sp. Not reliable or effective against other fungal pathogens	Caspofungin, anidulafungin insufficient data for prophylactic efficacy in pediatrics Micafungin shows superior efficacy compared to fluconazole as prophylaxis during neutropenia in HSCT recipients	In adults, 50 mg/day IV for prophylaxis No standardized pediatric dosing information for prophylaxis	Excellent safety profile

MDS myelodysplastic syndrome, *AML* acute myelogenous leukemia, *HSCT* hematopoietic stem cell transplant, *GVHD* graph versus host disease

[a]Amphotericin B formulations include: amphotericin B desoxycholate, liposomal amphotericin B (Ambisome®), amphotericin B lipid complex, and amphotericin B colloidal dispersion

Electrolyte Replacement

Children with malignancies can develop electrolyte imbalances due to the disease process or as a consequence of the associated therapy. Routine laboratory evaluations are necessary at the time of diagnosis and throughout treatment. Administration of oral or intravenous supplements may be needed to maintain normal electrolyte requirements. However, management of electrolytes is challenging during cancer therapy because of frequent changes in a patient's clinical condition and administration of multiple medications and fluids.

Routine oral magnesium supplementation is recommended with cisplatin-containing regimens, starting at a minimum of 6 mg (0.5 mEq) elemental magnesium/kg/day in divided doses [4]. For treatment of existing hypomagnesemia, use oral therapy of 20–40 mg elemental magnesium/kg/day in divided doses or intravenous therapy of 5–10 mg elemental magnesium/kg/dose (up to maximum of 250 mg elemental magnesium per IV dose) [10]. Some patients may require a continuous infusion of magnesium at a rate of 0.12 mmol magnesium/kg/day intravenously [10]. Use magnesium with caution in renal failure, and large doses may cause diarrhea (Table 14.5).

Granulocyte Colony-Stimulating Factor (G-CSF)

Hematopoietic growth-stimulating factors regulate the proliferation, differentiation, and function of hematopoietic cells [23]. Granulocyte colony-stimulating factor (G-CSF, filgrastim) and granulocyte–macrophage colony-stimulating factor (GM-CSF, sargramostim) have been effective in reducing the incidence of febrile neutropenia when initiated after chemotherapy or in bone marrow transplant patients [23]. G-CSF regulates the production of the neutrophil lineage, while GM-CSF stimulates the growth of granulocyte, macrophage, and eosinophil colonies [23]. The administration of both factors results in an increase of circulating neutrophils, thus decreasing the number and duration of febrile neutropenic episodes in both adults and children [24]. There is sufficient evidence that primary prophylaxis with colony-stimulating factors (CSFs) significantly reduces the relative risk of severe neutropenia, febrile neutropenia, and infection. There is insufficient evidence that CSFs reduce the number of patients requiring intravenous antibiotics, lower infection-related morbidity, or improve overall survival [25]. The available data also shows no difference in quality of life between placebo and CSF [25]. Further trials are required to compare the clinical activity, toxicity, and cost-effectiveness of G-CSF versus GM-CSF.

Table 14.5 Common electrolyte imbalances in pediatric oncology patients [2, 4, 10, 22]

Electrolyte imbalance	Etiology in oncology patients	Symptoms	Treatment
Hypercalcemia	Bone malignancies and metastases, poor dietary intake of phosphate, renal absorption or excretion, diuretics	GI (anorexia, nausea, vomiting, constipation, ileus) Neuromuscular (lethargy, apathy, depression, fatigue, hypotonia, stupor, coma) Cardiovascular (bradycardia, arrhythmia) Renal (polyuria, nocturia)	Hydration + diuretics Hemodialysis Steroids (i.e., predni- sone 1–2 mg/kg/ day) Correct underlying causes IV bisphosphonates (e.g., pamidronate)
Hypocalcemia	Reduced intake, vitamin D deficiency, intake or malabsorption; hypoparathyroidism, pancreatitis, cisplatin- induced renal tubular damage, tumor lysis syndrome	Neuromuscular irritability, weakness, cramping, fatigue, change in level of consciousness, seizures, ECG changes	Intravenous or oral calcium supplements Correct underlying causes IV calcium gluconate 50–100 mg/kg/dose (usual maximum of 3,000 mg/dose) or 0.1–0.2 mmol/kg/hr elemental calcium
Hyperkalemia	Renal failure, cellular breakdown (tumor lysis syndrome), leukocytosis, metabolic acidosis	ECG changes	Kayexalate (sodium polystyrene sulfonate 1 g/kg with 50% sorbitol) Insulin (0.1 units/ kg) + 25% dextrose (2 mL/kg) Sodium bicarbonate Calcium gluconate (100–200 mg/kg)
Hypokalemia	Decreased intake, increased renal excretion, therapy- induced renal tubular defects (i.e., ifosf- amide, cisplatin), diarrhea, vomiting, amphotericin formulations	Skeletal muscle weakness, dysrhythmias, prolonged QT interval, flattened T waves	Intravenous or oral potassium supplements 2–5 mmol/kg/day potassium oral or IV in divided doses

(continued)

Table 14.5 (continued)

Electrolyte imbalance	Etiology in oncology patients	Symptoms	Treatment
Hyponatremia	SIADH, ectopic secretion of antidiuretic hormone; renal, adrenal, cortical or cardiac insufficiency; excessive loss secondary to vomiting, diarrhea, nephropathy from ifosfamide, cyclophosphamide, or vinca alkaloids	Convulsions, shock, lethargy Headache, confusion, muscle cramping	Fluid restriction Replace sodium losses Correct underlying causes To correct acute, serious hyponatremia: mmol sodium – desired sodium (mmol/L) – actual sodium (mmol/L) times 0.6 times weight (kg)
Hypomagnesemia	Nephrotoxic agents (i.e., cisplatin-induced renal tubular damage, decreased intake, diarrhea, vomiting, urinary loss	Tetany, seizures, tremors, anorexia, nausea, cardiac abnormalities, weakness, clonus	Intravenous or oral magnesium supplements 1 mEq = 12 mg = 0.5 mMol (refer to paragraph below table)
Hypermagnesemia	Renal dysfunction	Hyporeflexia, respiratory depression, confusion, coma	Intravenous administration of calcium, diuresis
Hypophosphatemia	Poor dietary intake, malabsorption, excessive renal excretion, vitamin D deficiency, renal tubular damage from ifosfamide	Irritability, paresthesias	Intravenous or oral phosphate supplements Moderate (oral phosphate): 1–2 mmol/kg/day ÷ bid–qid Moderate–severe (IV phosphate therapy): 1–2 mmol/kg/day or 0.042–0.053 mmol/kg/hr
Hyperphosphatemia	Chemotherapy, renal insufficiency, glomerular filtration rate < 25% normal, tumor lysis syndrome	Symptoms same as with hypocalcemia	Restrict intake, phosphate binders (e.g., aluminum hydroxide), calcium supplements

SIADH syndrome of inappropriate antidiuretic hormone secretion

Recommendations for Use of CSFs in Pediatric Oncology Patients

Children with severe neutropenia (a reduction in the number of neutrophils that fight infection) are at risk of life-threatening infections (bacterial, fungal, and viral). The American Society of Clinical Oncology (ASCO) has published evidence-based clinical practice guidelines for the use of CSFs with the following recommendations for the pediatric population [25]:

1. The use of G-CSF in pediatric patients is usually guided by clinical protocols.
2. As in adults, the use of G-CSF is reasonable for the primary prophylaxis (to prevent myelosuppression) in patients at high risk of febrile neutropenia based on age, medical history, disease characteristics, and myelotoxicity of chemo-therapy regimen.
3. Use of G-CSF for secondary prophylaxis (to prevent new episodes of myelosup-pression in patients who experienced a neutropenic complication from a prior cycle of chemotherapy) should be limited to high-risk patients in which a reduced dose of chemotherapy or a delay may compromise survival or treatment outcome.
4. CSFs should not be routinely used as adjunctive treatment with antibiotic therapy for patients with fever and neutropenia but may be considered for patients at high risk for infection-related complications (e.g., expected prolonged neutropenia >10 days, uncontrolled primary disease, pneumonia, hypotension, multiorgan dysfunction, bacterial sepsis, invasive fungal infection).
5. In children with ALL (acute lymphoblastic leukemia), there is a potential risk for secondary myeloid leukemia or myelodysplastic syndrome (MDS) associated with G-CSF; therefore, prophylactic use of G-CSF is not recommended for patients with leukemia.

Dosing and Administration of CSFs

There is a theoretical risk that if CSFs are given concurrently with chemotherapy, they may induce progenitor cell cycling and cause increased myelotoxicity [1]. Therefore, it is recommended that G-CSF administration should begin 24–72 h after the administration of myelotoxic chemotherapy and continue through the period of granulocyte nadir until reaching an absolute neutrophil count (ANC) of at least $2-3 \times 10^9$/L [25]. The recommended dose of G-CSF is 5 mcg/kg/day, and the pre-ferred route of administration is subcutaneous, although it can be administered intravenously. The recommended dose for GM-CSF is 250 mcg/m^2/day.

Side Effects of CSFs

The predominant side effect reported with G-CSF is medullary bone pain (in 15–39% of patients) [2] which presents shortly after the injection or during the time of neutrophil recovery. This pain can be relieved by analgesics such as acetaminophen or nonsteroidal anti-inflammatory medications (e.g., ibuprofen, naproxen). Splenomegaly has been reported but is usually asymptomatic. Other infrequently reported adverse reactions include vasculitis, osteopenia, glomerulonephritis, rash, bone marrow fibrosis, anaphylaxis, and acute febrile neutropenic dermatosis (Sweet's syndrome). Worsening thrombocytopenia has also been observed with CSF administration in children [2].

Side effects are reported more frequently with GM-CSF and include fever, chills, lethargy, myalgia, bone pain, anorexia, generalized skin eruptions, weight changes, and flushing.

Menses Suppression (Therapeutic Amenorrhea)

Reproductive age female patients with thrombocytopenia are at increased risk of menorrhagia which can lead to significant blood loss requiring blood transfusions. Multiple transfusions put patients at risk for complications such as febrile non-hemolytic reactions, viral or bacterial infection, acute hemolytic reaction, anaphylactic reactions, volume and iron overload, etc. Thrombocytopenia may be disease-related (i.e., secondary to leukemia, myelodysplastic syndrome, aplastic anemia) or treatment induced by chemotherapy, radiation, or bone marrow transplantation. Therapeutic amenorrhea with pharmacologic agents should be considered in menstruating female cancer patients if they are experiencing or anticipating severe and prolonged thrombocytopenia. There are a number of effective hormonal regimens proposed to achieve therapeutic amenorrhea. The choice of method is dependent upon the patient's need for contraception and ability to tolerate estrogen-containing medications. Menses suppression is most effective when initiated before chemotherapy, radiation, or bone marrow transplant and prior to the development of thrombocytopenia [26]. Once initiated, suppression of menses should continue until the platelet count is ≥50,000/μ(micro)L without transfusion support [4]. Table 14.6 summarizes treatment options for therapeutic suppression of menses in patients at risk of thrombocytopenia.

In patients at an increased risk for venous thromboembolism, estrogen-containing methods should not be used. Estrogen-containing contraceptives are also contraindicated in patients with acute hepatoxicity and liver tumors. Progestin-only oral contraceptives or injectable progestins (Depo-Provera®) are safer options for these patients [26].

A major disadvantage of menstrual suppression is the increase in breakthrough bleeding that occurs during the first few cycles of using a hormonal method.

Table 14.6 Therapeutic options for menses suppression [26–29]

Method	Combined oral contraceptives (COCs)	Injectable progestin-only	Transdermal contraceptive patch	Levonorgestrel intrauterine device (IUD)	GnRH-a	Androgen therapy
Description and dosage	Low-dose monophasic, combined oral contraceptive pill; continued use (administration for unlimited time without interruption) required to eliminate menstrual periods (placebo week eliminated)	Depot medroxyprogesterone acetate (DMPA) 150 mg intramuscular injection every 12 weeks	For extended use, replace patch every week without a patch-free interval Releases 150 mcg norelgestromin + 20 mcg ethinyl estradiol daily	Progestin-releasing IUD Releases 20 mg of levonorgestrel daily; effective for 5 years	Gonadotropin-releasing hormone agonist;delivery methods and dosages vary (intramuscular depot or intravenous injections or intranasally)	Gonadotropin inhibitor with progestational and androgenic properties; 100–200 mg twice daily oral
Contraception provided	Yes	Yes	Yes	Yes	No	No
Efficacy in ↓ blood loss	Induces progressive endometrial atrophy Continuous use eliminates menstrual periods in 53% of women by 1 year of use	Induces endometrial atrophy; amenorrhea uncommon in first few months but common with long-term use (55–60% after 1 yr; 90% after 2 yrs)	Studies not published but regimens similar to COCs suppress menstruation	80–90% decrease in blood loss; ~20% of users are amenorrheic by 1 year of use	Requires 2–4 weeks to induce amenorrhea; superior to DMPA in suppressing hypermenorrhea in patients receiving myelosuppressive therapy	In refractory ITP patients, 84% had amenorrhea or oligomenorrhea after 1–2 months treatment

(continued)

Table 14.6 (continued)

Method	Combined oral contraceptives (COCs)	Injectable progestin-only	Transdermal contraceptive patch	Levonorgestrel intrauterine device (IUD)	GnRH-a	Androgen therapy
Adverse effects	Safety of continuous use comparable to conventional COC regimens, although breakthrough bleeding can occur Intrahepatic cholestasis uncommon (idiosyncratic reaction) ↑ Risk of venous thromboembolism (VTE) 3–4 fold (highest risk in first year of use)	High incidence of breakthrough bleeding and spotting Significant loss of bone mineral density with longer duration of use Possible weight gain Delayed return to fertility Headache, nausea	Possible incidence of venous thromboembolism (VTE) Headaches, local skin irritation (20%), nausea, abdominal pain	Breakthrough bleeding, ovarian cysts, acne Risk of IUD-associated pelvic inflammatory disease during first 20 days post insertion	Main effects are severe bone loss (3% over 3 months) and unfavorable lipid profile; menopausal symptoms (i.e., vaginal dryness, hot flushes) significant bleeding more likely if given <2 weeks before development of thrombocytopenia (decreased success if thrombocytopenia has already occurred)	Androgenic effects limit use (i.e., weight gain, acne, asthenia, myalgias, partial hair loss, headaches); hypoestrogenic reactions (i.e., flushing, sweating, vaginal dryness, irritation)

Place in therapy for pediatric oncology patients	Preferred method by COG as treatment of choice if no concern about estrogen or patient compliance. Compliance compromised by nausea, emesis, mucositis, or elevated bilirubin related to chemotherapy	Second line if estrogen containing COCs are not an option	Alternative to oral COCs in patients who cannot tolerate oral medications or if compliance with COCs a concern. Okay for use with liver tumors, hepatotoxicity	Not usually considered for neutropenic or immunosuppressed patients because of infection risk. Literature on IUD usage in immunosuppressed women is extremely limited	Not practical for acute effect given the 2–4 week delay in amenorrhea; best suited for perimenopausal women for short time frame	Not first line because of androgenic side effects
Cost	Low cost	Low cost	Slightly more expensive than COCs	Initial high cost; cost-effective with extended use	Very expensive	Expensive
Examples	Alesse-28®	Depo-Provera®	Ortho Evra®	Mirena®	Leuprolide acetate (Lupron Depot®)	Danazol®

COCs combination oral contraceptives, *COG* Children's Oncology Group

For example, breakthrough bleeding is common after the initial dose of depo-medroxyprogesterone acetate, and this can be managed by reducing the dosing interval to every 2 months or supplementing with a high-dose estrogen COC for 1–3 months. However, the high-dose estrogen will lead to endometrial growth, and once the estrogen therapy is stopped, the patient is at risk of an estrogen withdrawal bleed. Consultation with a gynecologist is recommended prior to initiating therapeutic amenorrhea or when problematic bleeding occurs (Table 14.6).

References

1. Panzarella C, Baggott CR, Comeau M, et al. Management of disease and treatment-related complications. In: Baggott CR, Kelly KP, Fochtman D, Foley GV, eds. Nursing Care of Children and Adolescents with Cancer. 3rd ed. Philadelphia, Pa: W.B. Wanders Company;2002:279–318.
2. Berde CB, Billett AL, Collins JJ. Symptom management in supportive care. In: Pizzo PA, Poplack DG, eds. Principles and Practice of Pediatric Oncology. 4th ed. Philadelphia, Pa: Lippincott Williams & Wilkins;2002:1301–1332.
3. Antonarakis ES, Hain RDW. Nausea and vomiting associated with cancer chemotherapy: drug management in theory and in practice. Archives of Disease in Childhood. 2004;89:877–880.
4. Children's Oncology Group Supportive Care Guidelines. https://members.childrensoncology-group.org/_files/protocol/standard/SupportiveCareGuidelines.pdf. Accessed November 29, 2010.
5. Cancer Care Ontario: Management of chemotherapy-induced nausea and vomiting. http://www.cancercare.on.ca. Accessed February 1, 2010.
6. Policy for the treatment of chemotherapy induced nausea and vomiting. http://www.yorkshire-cancer-net.org.uk/html/downloads/ycn_hyccn_cyp_haematology_oncology_chemotherapyin-ducednauseaandvomiting_dec2009.pdf. Accessed December 11, 2010.
7. Dupuis LL, Nathan PC. Optimizing emetic control in children receiving antineoplastic therapy. Pediatric Drugs. 2010;12(1):51–61.
8. Kris MG, Hesketh PJ, Somerfield MR, et al. American Society of Clinical Oncology guideline for antiemetics in oncology: Update 2006. Journal of Clinical Oncology. 2006;24(16):2932–2947.
9. FDA Drug Safety Communication - Abnormal heart rhythms associated with the use of Anzemet (dolasetron mesylate). http://www.fda.gov/Drugs/DrugSafety/ucm237081.htm. Accessed December 21, 2010.
10. Lau E, ed. The Hospital for Sick Children 2009–2010 Drug Handbook and Formulary. Toronto, ON.
11. Prasad P, Nania JJ, Shankar SM. Pneumocystis pneumonia in children receiving chemotherapy. Pediatric Blood & Cancer. 2008;50:896–898.
12. Kim SY, Dabb AA, Glenn DJ, et al. Intravenous pentamidine is effective as second line pneumocystis pneumonia prophylaxis in pediatric oncology patients. Pediatric Blood & Cancer. 2008;50:779–783.
13. CDC: Guidelines for prophylaxis against pneumocystis carinii pneumonia for children infected with human immunodeficiency virus. http://www.cdc.gov/mmwr/preview/mmwrhtml/00001957.htm. Accessed January 12, 2011.
14. Williams S, MacDonald P, Hoyer JD, et al. Methemoglobinemia in children with acute lymphoblastic leukemia (ALL) receiving dapsone for pneumocystis carinii pneumonia (PCP) prophylaxis: A correlation with cytochrome b5 reductase (CB5R) enzyme levels. Cancer. 2005;44:55–62.

15. Chuk MK, Dabb AA, Kim SY, et al. The use of IV pentamidine as second line prophylaxis for pneumocystis pneumonia. Journal of Clinical Oncology. 2006 ASCO Annual Meeting Proceedings Part I;24(18 S):9043.
16. PCP prophylaxis: What to do when SMX/TMS fails? http://www.isopp.org/files/education.../ Rao%20PCP%20Prophylxais%20Final.pdf. Accessed February 26, 2011.
17. Pneumocystis carinii pneumonia. http://www.medicine.gerogetown.edu/residency/BoardReview/ PCP.PPT. Accessed February 26, 2011.
18. Robenshtok E, Gafter-Gvili A, Goldberg E, et al. Antifungal prophylaxis in cancer patients after chemotherapy or hematopoietic stem-cell transplantation: Systematic review and meta-analysis. Journal of Clinical Oncology. 2007;25:5471–5489.
19. Bow EJ, Laverdiere M, Lussier N, et al. Antifungal prophylaxis for severely neutropenic chemotherapy patients. Cancer. 2002;94:3230–3246.
20. Groll AH, Just-Nuebling G, Kurz M, et al. Fluconazole versus nystatin in the prevention of candida infections in children and adolescents undergoing remission induction or consolidation chemotherapy for cancer. Journal of Antimicrobial Chemotherapy. 1997;40:855–862.
21. NCCN Practice guidelines in oncology: Prevention and treatment of cancer-related infections. http://www.oralcancerfoundationorg./treatment/pdf/infections-NCCN.pdf. Accessed February 26, 2011.
22. Rodgers C, Gonzalez S. Nutrition and hydration in children with cancer. In: Tomlinson D, Kline NE, eds. Pediatric Oncology Nursing: Advanced Clinical Handbook. 2nd ed. New York, NY: Springer-Verlag Berlin Heidelberg;2010:515–528.
23. Clark OAC, Lyman GH, Castro AA, et al. Colony-stimulating factors for chemotherapy-induced febrile neutropenia: A meta-analysis of randomized controlled trials. Journal of Clinical Oncology. 2005;23(18):4198–4214.
24. Bukowski R. Cytoprotection in the treatment of pediatric cancer: Review of current strategies in adults and their application to children. Medical and Pediatric Oncology. 1999;32:124–134.
25. Smith TJ, Khatcheressian J, Lyman GH, et al. 2006 Update of recommendations for the use of white blood cell growth factors: An evidence-based clinical practice guideline. Journal of Clinical Oncology. 2006;24(19):3187–3205.
26. Martin-Johnston MK, Okoji OY, Armstrong A. Therapeutic amenorrhea in patients at risk for thrombocytopenia. Obstetrical and Gynecological Survey. 2008;63(6):395–401.
27. Extended and continuous use of contraceptives to reduce menstruation. http://www.arhp.org/ Publications-and-Resources/Clinical-Proceedings/Reduce-Menses. Accessed January 12, 2011.
28. Fisher WA, Black A. Contraception in Canada: A review of method choices, characteristics, adherence and approaches to counseling. CMAJ. 2007;176(7):953–961.
29. Hillard PJA. Therapeutic amenorrhea. Journal of Pediatric Hematology/Oncology. 1999;21(5): 350–352.

Chapter 15
Abdominal Complications

Hanna Tseitlin

Keywords Antibiotic coverage • Asparaginase • Bowel ischemia • Constipation • Enemas • Fecal loading • Hematochezia • Mucosal injury • Neutropenic entero-colitis • Pancreatitis • Peritonitis • Pneumatosis intestinalis • Typhlitis

Introduction

The gastrointestinal system is often a target of toxicity of chemotherapy due to its natural pattern of rapid cell division. Different treatment modalities such as chemotherapy, radiation, and surgery as well as underlying disease processes are known to alter the mucosal surface and lead to life-threatening complications. Mucosal injury and destruction increase permeability of the mucosal barrier and lead to edema, inflammation, and bacterial invasion. Consequently, it may trigger intestinal perforation, peritonitis, sepsis, and death.

The most common gastrointestinal complications in children undergoing chemotherapy and radiotherapy treatments are constipation, typhlitis, pneumatosis, and pancreatitis. Some of the clinical symptoms overlap and make the differential diagnosis difficult (Table 15.1).

H. Tseitlin (✉)
Division of Hematology/Oncology, McMaster Children's Hospital,
1280 Main Street West, Hamilton, ON, Canada L8S 4K1
e-mail: tseitlin@hhsc.ca

K. Scheinemann and A.E. Boyce (eds.), *Emergencies in Pediatric Oncology*,
DOI 10.1007/978-1-4614-1174-1_15, © Springer Science+Business Media, LLC 2012

Constipation

Definition

Constipation is often difficult to define due to its subjective symptomatology and dependence on an individual's elimination habits. The signs of constipation may include abdominal fullness, bloating, hard stools, abdominal cramping, and difficulty defecating.

Causes of constipation, as with other gastrointestinal complications, are often multifactorial in children undergoing treatment for malignant diseases. It may be related to lack of mobility, dietary choices, dehydration due to fluid loss, and bowel obstruction due to disease process. The administration of some chemotherapeutic agents, such as vincristine, or medications such as antiemetics and opiates may also result in constipation.

Despite complexities in its definition and the subjective nature of bowel elimination habits, there are guidelines that define acceptable elimination patterns for children of different ages. Younger children usually have more frequent bowel movements; however, as they get older, the frequency decreases and does not change after the age of 4 years. Children 4 years of age or older should have anywhere between 3 and 14 bowel movements per week.

Some of the subjective signs associated with constipation are general irritability and abdominal cramps that are often described by children as abdominal pain and decreased oral intake. Other signs may include vomiting and abdominal distention [1]. Changes in personal elimination habits related to frequency and quantity of stool should be taken into account when establishing the diagnosis of constipation [2].

Prevalence and Diagnosis

Prevalence of constipation in healthy children has been reported anywhere between 2% and 10%; however, in children undergoing chemotherapy treatment, the prevalence has been reported to be as high as 50–100% [2–4].

The diagnosis of constipation is primarily based on medical history and physical examination although some radiological investigations could be useful. Plain X-ray can easily identify fecal loading, having been shown to have a detection sensitivity of 92% and specificity of 62% [1]. Since children undergoing chemotherapy treatment have an increased risk for developing gastrointestinal complications with similar presentations, the diagnosis of constipation is often based on exclusion of other conditions.

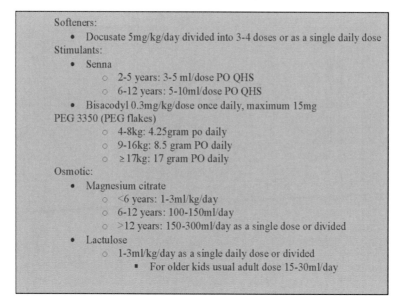

Softeners:
- Docusate 5mg/kg/day divided into 3-4 doses or as a single daily dose

Stimulants:
- Senna
  - 2-5 years: 3-5 ml/dose PO QHS
  - 6-12 years: 5-10ml/dose PO QHS
- Bisacodyl 0.3mg/kg/dose once daily, maximum 15mg

PEG 3350 (PEG flakes)
  - 4-8kg: 4.25gram po daily
  - 9-16kg: 8.5 gram PO daily
  - ≥17kg: 17 gram PO daily

Osmotic:
- Magnesium citrate
  - <6 years: 1-3ml/kg/day
  - 6-12 years: 100-150ml/day
  - >12 years: 150-300ml/day as a single dose or divided
- Lactulose
  - 1-3ml/kg/day as a single daily dose or divided
    - For older kids usual adult dose 15-30ml/day

Fig. 15.1 Bowel regimen medications and dosages

Management

The key to managing constipation in children undergoing chemotherapy treatment is prevention. Therefore, bowel regimens should be introduced soon after starting chemotherapy protocols, as outlined in Fig. 15.1. Prior to initiating treatment for constipation, a thorough physical examination should be administered and blood counts assessed. Enemas and suppositories are contraindicated in children undergoing chemotherapy due to risk of infection and perforation, especially in the presence of neutropenia. Exception could be made with those children who are not neutropenic at the time of assessment for constipation.

Definition of Typhlitis

Typhlitis, also referred to as neutropenic enterocolitis, is a constellation of symptoms often observed in patients undergoing chemotherapy treatments. The symptoms include abdominal pain, fever, abdominal distention, and diminished bowel sounds. Neutropenia is the most common laboratory finding for the majority of patients.

It was first described in 1970 and was initially attributed to the complication of childhood leukemia. It was subsequently recognized as a potentially life-threatening complication in children and adults undergoing treatments for both hematological and solid malignancies as well as in patients with AIDS, aplastic anemia, MDS, and those undergoing bone marrow transplant [5–7].

Table 15.1 Diagnostic workup for severe abdominal pain

Diagnostic workup:
- History
- Physical examination
- Blood work
  - CBC
  - Chemistry
    - Electrolytes
    - Urea
    - Creatinine
    - Albumin
    - Total protein
    - Liver functions
  - Blood cultures
    - From central line; both lumens if a double-lumen catheter is present
    - Peripheral
- Stool samples for *Clostridium difficile*
- Radiological investigations
  - Abdominal X-ray
  - Abdominal ultrasound
  - Abdominal CT – reserve for cases when other modalities were inconclusive

Typhlitis is defined as the inflammatory process of the cecum; however, it may also involve terminal ileum and ascending colon. It is described as bowel wall thickening with inflammation, edema, and mucosal ulceration and necrosis [8–10]. The etiology of typhlitis is not clearly defined. Believed to be multifactorial, it entails mucosal destruction and injury that leads to a loss of barrier in face of gastrointestinal microorganisms, neutropenia that supports microbial invasion, as well as intramural hemorrhages related to thrombocytopenia and subsequent inflammation, edema, and necrosis [10, 11].

Prevalence and Diagnosis

The incidence of typhlitis in children undergoing chemotherapy treatment for either leukemia/lymphoma or solid tumors has been reported to be 3 and 2.5%, respectively [6, 11]. The diagnostic workup should include a thorough medical history, physical examination, laboratory workup, and radiological investigations.

History findings may include complaints of abdominal pain, fever, diarrhea, and vomiting. Constipation is present in about 6% of patients, and hematochezia has been reported in about 25% of the patients. Physical findings often include abdominal tenderness on palpation, localized to the right lower quadrant, and abdominal distention [12]. In view of the fact that typhlitis is often referred to as neutropenic enterocolitis, the most common laboratory finding associated with typhlitis is neutropenia, defined as neutrophil count of less than 500 cells/μL. Other laboratory findings may include anemia and thrombocytopenia and electrolyte disturbances such as hypokalemia, hypophosphatemia, and hypoalbuminemia. Blood cultures

Table 15.2 Nonsurgical management of typhlitis

Non surgical management of typhlitis:
• Bowel rest – NPO until symptoms' resolution
• Total parenteral nutrition support
• Fluid resuscitation
• Broad-spectrum antibiotic coverage as per institutional febrile/neutropenia guidelines
• Adjust antibiotic coverage based on sensitivity in the presence of positive cultures
• Nasogastric suctioning
• Correction of electrolyte abnormalities
• Continuous narcotics infusion for severe abdominal pain

are positive in about 25% of cases with *E. coli*, Pseudomonas species, Klebsiella species, and viridans group streptococci.

Radiological findings may include bowel wall thickening, accumulation of paracolonic fluid, free air, and pneumatosis intestinalis [7, 12].

Management

The management of typhlitis is based on supportive medical measures, with surgical interventions reserved for severe cases with a presence of perforation, sepsis, peritonitis, gangrenous bowel, and persistent gastrointestinal hemorrhage. Supportive medical measures include bowel rest, nutritional support with TPN, antimicrobials, and nasogastric suctioning [8, 11, 12] (Table 15.2).

Definition of Pneumatosis Intestinalis

Pneumatosis intestinalis (PI) is defined as air within the bowel wall and is most commonly present in premature infants as a sign of bowel ischemia. Its occurrence decreases in children older than 1 year of age and is rarely observed in adults. Children undergoing chemotherapy treatment face an increased risk of developing PI as a result of destruction of bowel mucosa and increased permeability of the gut. The etiology of PI is unknown; however, several hypotheses have been proposed to include mucosal injury and increased permeability with gas diffusion from the bowel lumen into the bowel wall, bacterial invasion with intramural gas production, and increased intraluminal pressure facilitating gas diffusion. PI typically occurs in the colon, most commonly in the ascending and transverse segments; however, in some cases, it has also been reported in the terminal ileum [13, 14]. Approximately 5–10% of patients with PI could be asymptomatic and are diagnosed incidentally on plain abdominal radiographs when investigating for other conditions. When symptomatic, children often present with abdominal pain, abdominal distention, vomiting, and constipation; fever and neutropenia are often

Table 15.3 Nonsurgical management of PI

Non surgical management of PI:
- Bowel rest – NPO until symptom resolution
- Total parenteral nutrition support
- Fluid resuscitation
- Broad-spectrum antibiotic coverage as per institutional febrile/neutropenia guidelines
  - Adjust antibiotic coverage based on sensitivity in the presence of positive cultures
- Nasogastric suctioning
- Continuous narcotics infusion for pain control
- Surgical consultation

found at the time of presentation. A more severe presentation of PI has been attributed to perforation resulting in pneumoperitoneum, peritonitis, and sepsis [13, 14].

Prevalence and Diagnosis

Intensive chemotherapy protocols such as treatments for acute myeloid leukemia (AML) and use of steroids for the induction of acute lymphoblastic leukemia (ALL) have been strongly associated with incidents of PI in the pediatric oncology population. Chemotherapeutic agents such as vincristine, asparaginase, methotrexate, and cytarabine have been implicated as possible causes when received 30 days prior to development of PI. Since these agents are most commonly used for treatment of ALL and AML, the prevalence rate of PI in that population is 4–5% [14].

Plain abdominal radiographs are adequate for identifying PI in majority of children and are sufficient for making a diagnosis. In cases where the results of plain X-ray cannot definitively confirm the presence of PI, abdominal CT should be utilized to confirm the diagnosis. Since abdominal ultrasounds identify only 20% of PI cases, they should not be used for diagnostic purposes [14, 15].

Management

As with typhlitis, conservative medical management should be implemented in the absence of peritonitis and sepsis (Table 15.3).

Definition of Pancreatitis

Pancreatitis is defined as an inflammatory process of the pancreas and is often described in association with asparaginase treatment for ALL in pediatric oncology patients. Other chemotherapy agents that have been associated with acute pancreatitis are ifosphamide, 6-mercaptopurine, and vinca alkaloids; however, those cases are

Table 15.4 Pancreatitis [17–20]

Clinical symptoms of acute pancreatitis	Laboratory findings of acute pancreatitis	Radiological findings
Abdominal pain and irritability	Serum amylase >3× ULN	Pancreatic enlargement
Nausea and/or vomiting	Lipase >1.5× ULN	Free fluid in the abdominal cavity
Epigastric tenderness		Loss of pancreatic contours and/or pseudocyst

rarely seen [16]. Since leukemia is the most common malignancy in childhood, and asparaginase is an important component of the leukemic protocol, asparaginase-associated acute pancreatitis should be examined in this part.

Prevalence and Diagnosis

The prevalence of acute pancreatitis has been reported to be between 2 and 18% in children undergoing treatment for ALL. This wide variation in incidence has been related to the difference in administration protocols and asparaginase preparation [17–19]. Children older than 10 years of age at the time of ALL diagnosis have twofold higher incidence of pancreatitis when compared to younger children [18].

The diagnosis of pancreatitis is based on clinical symptoms and laboratory abnormalities, as well as radiological findings. Abdominal pain has been identified as the key clinical feature with 100% of patients exhibiting the symptom. Irritability, nausea, and vomiting have been reported in about 75% of cases [20]. Some patients may have a concurrent febrile neutropenic episode; however, it is usually unrelated to the diagnosis of acute pancreatitis.

Abdominal ultrasound is the most commonly used modality for confirming a clinically suspicious case of acute pancreatitis. However, it must be noted that in some children evaluated with abdominal ultrasound, acute pancreatitis is not always detected despite the presence of clinical and laboratory findings. Abdominal CT should be reserved for children exhibiting worsening or persistence of symptoms. It should also be considered in children that present with the clinical picture of acute pancreatitis and nondiagnostic ultrasound (Table 15.4).

Management

Pancreatitis is usually managed conservatively, with surgery reserved for managing complications such as pseudocyst.

Antibiotic coverage should only be implemented when concurrent fever and neutropenia are present. Nutritional intake could be introduced with resolution of symptoms and improvement in pancreatic enzymes and should follow a progressive schedule from clear fluids to full diet as tolerated by the child. In the event of

Table 15.5 Pancreatitis management

Pancreatitis management:
- Pain control with intravenous narcotics
- Bowel rest
- Nasogastric tube and gastric suctioning
- Total parenteral nutrition support
- Daily enzyme follow-up
Surgical team referral

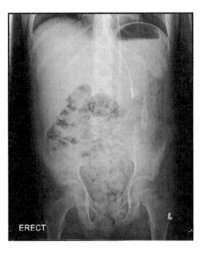

Fig. 15.2 Abdominal X-ray revealed invasive fecal loading in the colon

recurrence of symptoms and rebound elevation of pancreatic enzymes while advancing the diet, bowel rest should be reintroduced until new improvement is evident. Subsequent progression of the diet could be initiated as tolerated (Table 15.5).

Summary

Gastrointestinal complications in children undergoing chemotherapy treatments are multifactorial and require a systemic approach. Thorough history and physical examination should be obtained in a child presenting with abdominal discomfort. Underlying diagnosis and chemotherapeutic agents should be taken into account when establishing differential diagnosis. A high index of suspicion should be present while examining children with subtle abdominal symptoms, since those could be blunted by neutropenia and steroid administration, masking a gastrointestinal emergency. While conservative treatments are preferred for managing gastrointestinal complications, a surgical team should be consulted to evaluate the need for surgical interventions.

Case 1   Constipation
A 14-year-old boy with underlying pelvic Ewing's sarcoma and neurogenic bladder/bowel complains of severe back pain through clinic visits. He reports regular bowel movements (Fig. 15.2).

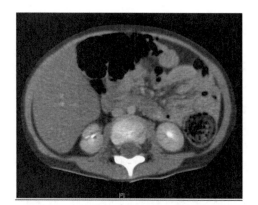

Fig. 15.3 Abdominal CT

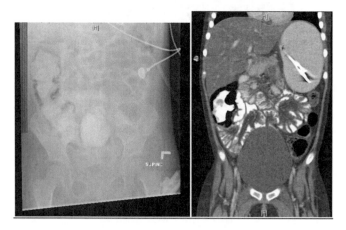

Fig. 15.4 Abdominal X-ray and CT scan

Case 2   Typhlitis
A four-and-a-half-year-old girl with underlying history of ALL presents with neutropenia and severe abdominal pain. Abdominal CT shows gas-filled fusiform bowel loops in the left abdomen. A few bubbles are seen below the abdominal wall which are concerning for extraluminal bubbles (Fig. 15.3).

Case 3   Pneumatosis
An almost 5-year-old girl with underlying history of ALL presents with neutropenia and severe abdominal pain. Abdominal X-ray and CT reveal pneumatosis in the ascending colon (Fig. 15.4).

Case 4   Pancreatitis
An almost 6-year-old boy treated with asparaginase for underlying ALL. He presented with decreased oral intake, severe lower abdominal pain, and emesis. Pancreatic enzymes were done: peak amylase was 169 U/L, peak lipase was 1334 U/L.

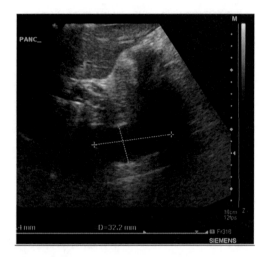

Fig. 15.5 Abdominal ultrasound

Abdominal ultrasound revealed a hypoechoic area at the pancreas measuring
$9.8 \times 6.7 \times 3.2$ cm, highly suggestive of a pancreatic pseudocyst (Fig. 15.5).

References

1. Baker, S.S., Liptak, G.S., Colletti, R.B., Croffie, J.M., Di Lorenzo, C., Ector, W. and Nurko, S. Evaluation and treatment of constipation in infants and children: recommendations of the North American Society for Pediatric Gastroenterology, Hepatology and Nutrition. Journal of Pediatric Gastroenterology and Nutrition. 2006; 43, e1-e13.
2. Woorley, M., Carroll, E., Fenn, E., Wieland, H., Jarosinski, P., Corey, B. and Wallen, G.R. A constipation assessment scale for use in pediatric oncology. Journal of Pediatric Oncology Nursing. 2006;23, pp.65-74
3. Mugie, S.M. and Benninga, M.A Epidemiology of constipation in children and adults: A systematic review. Best Practice and Research Clinical Gastroenterology. 2011; 25, pp.3-18
4. Selwood, K. Constipation in pediatric oncology. European Journal of Oncology Nursing. 2006; 10, pp.68-70
5. McCarville, M.B., Thompson, J., Li, C., Adelman, C.S., Lee, M.O., Alsammarae, D., May, M.V., Jones, S.C., Rao, B.N. and Sandlund, J.T. Significance of appendiceal thickening in association with typhlitis in pediatric oncology patients. Pediatric Radiology. 2004; 34, pp.245-249
6. McCarville, M.B., Adelman, C.S., Li, C., Xiong, X., Furman, W.L., Razzouk, B.I., Pui, C.-H. and Sandlund, J.T. Typhlitis in childhood cancer. Cancer. 2005;104(2), pp. 380–387
7. Moran, H., Yaniv, I., Ashkenazi, S., Schwartz, M., Fisher, S. and Levy, I. Risk factors for typhlitis in pediatric patients with cancer. Journal of Pediatric Hematology Oncology. 2009; 31(9), pp. 630–634
8. Gray, T.L.V., Ooi, C.Y., Tran, D., Traubici, J., Gerstle, J.T. and Sung, L. Gastrointestinal complications in children with acute myeloid leukemia. Leukemia and Lymphoma. 2010; 51(5), pp.768-777
9. Mullassery, D., Bader, A., Battersby, A.J., Mohammad, Z., Jones, E.L.L., Parmar, C., Scott, R., Pizer, B.L. and Baillie, C.T. Diagnosis, incidence and outcomes of suspected typhlitis in oncology

patients- experience in a tertiary pediatric surgical center in the United Kingdom. Journal of Pediatric Surgery. 2009; 44, pp.381-385

10. Van de Wetering, M.D., Kuijpers, T.W., Taminiau, J.A.J.M., ten Kate, F.J.W. and Caron, H.N. Pseudomembranous and neutropenic enterocolitis in pediatric oncology patients. Supportive Care in Cancer. 2003; 11, pp. 581–586

11. Ullery, B.W., Pieracci, F.M., Rodney, J.R.M. and Barie, P.S. Neutropenic enterocolitis. Surgical Infections. 2009; 10(3), pp.307-314

12. Schlatter, M., Snyder, K., and Freyer, D. Successful nonoperative management of typhlitis in pediatric oncology patients. Journal of Pediatric Surgery. 2002; 37(8), pp. 1151–1155

13. Groninger, E., Hulscher, J.B.F., Timmer, B., Tamminga, R.Y.J. and Broens, P.M.A. Free air intraperitoneally during chemotherapy for acute lymphoblastic leukemia: consider pneumatosis cystoides intestinalis. Journal of Pediatric Hematology Oncollogy. 2010; 32, pp.141-143

14. Li, S., Traubici, J., Ethier, M.-C., Gillmeister, B., Alexander, S., Gassass, A. and Sung, L. Pneumatosis intestinalis in children with acute lymphoblastic leukemia and acute myeloid leukemia. Supportive Care in Cancer. 2011; ahead of print.

15. Fenton L.Z. and Buonomo, C. Benign pneumatosis in children. Pediatric Radiology. 2000; 30, pp. 786–793

16. Garg, R., Agarwala, S. and Bhatnagar, V. Acute pancreatitis induced by ifosfamide therapy. Journal of Pediatric Surgery. 2010; 45, pp.2071-2073

17. Treepongkaruna, S., Thongpak, N., Pakakasama, S., Pienvichit, P., Sirachainan, N. and Hongeng, S. Acute pancreatitis in children with acute lymphoblastic leukemia after chemotherapy. Journal of Pediatric Hematology Oncology. 2009; 31(11), pp. 812–815

18. Kerney, S.L., Dahlberg, S.E., Levy, D.E., Voss, S.D., Sallan, S.E., and Silverman, L.B. Clinical course and outcome in children with acute lymphoblastic leukemia and asparaginase-associated pancreatitis. Pediatric Blood and Cancer. 2009; 53, pp.162-167

19. Knoderer, H.M., Robarge, J. and Flockhart, D.A. Predicting asparaginase-associated pancreatitis. Pediatric Blood and Cancer. 2007; 49, pp. 634–639

20. Park, A.J., Latif, S.U., Ahmad, M.U., Bultron, G., Orabi, A.I., Bhandari, V. and Hussain, S.Z. A comparison of presentation and management trends in acute pancreatitis between infants/toddlers and older children. Journal of Gastroenterology and Nutrition. 2010; 51(2), pp. 167–170

Chapter 16
Emergency Radiation Therapy in Pediatric Oncology

Laurence Masson-Côté, David C. Hodgson, Barbara-Ann Millar, and Normand J. Laperriere

Keywords Abdominal masses • Acute radiation reactions • Hepatomegaly • High-dose dexamethasone • High-energy photons • Hyperfractionated regimens • Inferior vena cava obstruction • Intensity-modulated radiation therapy (IMRT) • Mediastinal masses • Musculoskeletal toxicity • Myelopathy • Parallel-opposed technique • Scoliosis • Spinal cord compression • Spinal instability • Superior vena cava syndrome

Introduction

There are few but distinct emergency situations where radiation therapy (RT) is indicated in pediatric oncology. Radiotherapy can provide a highly effective noninvasive option for local and locoregional response, supporting the use of this modality in clinical circumstances where rapid decompression of critical structures is needed and surgery is not warranted.

Principles of Radiation Therapy

High-energy photons have no mass or electrical charge, but as they travel in tissue, they randomly strip electrons from atoms. As water is the commonest molecule in biologic tissues, most of the effects of ionizing radiation are by creating a hydroxy radical by stripping an electron from a water molecule, a highly reactive molecule

L. Masson-Côté • D.C. Hodgson • B.-A. Millar • N.J. Laperriere (✉)
Department of Radiation Oncology, Princess Margaret Hospital,
610 University Avenue, Toronto, ON, Canada M5G 2M9
e-mail: Norm.Laperriere@rmp.uhn.on.ca

K. Scheinemann and A.E. Boyce (eds.), *Emergencies in Pediatric Oncology*,
DOI 10.1007/978-1-4614-1174-1_16, © Springer Science+Business Media, LLC 2012

which will interact with the DNA of the cell and result in either a single- or double-stranded DNA break. Double-strand breaks may lead to chromosomal aberrations, and eventually to cell death, mainly during mitosis, when the cell attempts to divide. Because most of the cell death caused by radiation occurs when cells attempt to divide, one sees the effects of radiotherapy at various time intervals following radiation exposure, largely governed by the kinetics of the different tissues exposed. This explains why mucosal surface reactions (mucositis of oropharynx, diarrhea with bowel radiation, skin erythema, and hair loss) tend to be acute effects seen within weeks of beginning radiation, whereas subcutaneous fibrosis, growth, and vascular changes tend to be months to years following radiation exposure [1, 2].

Significant technological advances in radiation oncology have been made in the recent decade. Treatment planning now commonly employs 3D computed tomography (CT), magnetic resonance (MR), and positron emission tomography (PET) imaging, whereas previously only 2D imaging was available. An optimal dose to target can now be delivered with minimal dose to normal structures using 3D conformal radiation therapy or, when available, intensity-modulated radiation therapy (IMRT). Also, image-guided radiation therapy (IGRT), notably illustrated by the use cone beam CT imaging on treatment units to ensure the accurate positioning of the patient prior to treatment, has tremendously improved the precision of radiation delivery, reducing the margin of error to below 1 mm in many settings.

Mediastinal Masses

Mediastinal masses causing superior vena cava syndrome or acute airway compromise are one of the indications for emergency radiation therapy in the pediatric population. This presentation occurs mainly in association with lymphoma, and less commonly with sarcoma and neuroblastoma. Emergency RT for lymphoma patients is only provided when chemotherapy is contraindicated due to severe hemodynamic instability or other organ failure. More often, the first cycle of chemotherapy can produce a rapid response and symptomatic relief.

Details of the differential diagnosis, investigation, and therapy options associated to mediastinal masses in children are presented in Chap. 4. The following text focuses only on the aspects of emergency RT in this context. It is important to note that a biopsy should always be obtained if possible prior to treatment since RT can interfere with histologic diagnosis [3].

Rationale and Evidence

For decades, the efficacy of radiation therapy to relieve mediastinal compression secondary to tumor masses has been recognized [4]. Many publications in adult patients with superior vena cava syndrome, mainly secondary to lung cancer, have repeatedly shown an excellent response rate to emergency irradiation in the order of 75–80% [5–7].

Similar data in the pediatric literature are rare. Bertsch et al. published in 1998 the experience of the Children's Hospital of Philadelphia in terms of urgent thera-peutic irradiation in pediatric oncology from 1988 to 1994 [8]. In their cohort of 104 patients, 18 presented with respiratory compromise, the majority (12) due to a medi-astinal mass. The response rate to radiotherapy was 72%.

Technique

Planning procedures depend on the severity of the respiratory compromise. If the supine position can be tolerated, CT images should be obtained to allow a 3D or IMRT conformal irradiation. If CT planning is impossible, bony landmarks and a clinical markup can be used for a simple parallel-opposed pair technique. However, as soon as the child's clinical condition allows it, a conformal technique should be used to deliver the remaining treatments. Usually 1.5–2 Gy per fraction to a total dose of 6–7.5 Gy should be adequate to relieve symptoms. Hyperfractionated regi-mens (1.2–1.5 Gy per fraction twice a day to a total dosage of to 10 Gy) are another option [9].

Expected Side Effects with Recommended Doses/Fractionations

Expected side effects with the recommended dose and technique are low as detailed in Table 16.1. Since this treatment is often offered in a palliative setting, late effects may not be of substantial clinical concern.

Case 1

This 8-year-old boy with recurrent Ewing's sarcoma presented with a significant progression of a known metastatic mediastinal mass and secondary marked com-pression of his trachea (Figs. 16.1 and 16.2).

This patient was also known with other extrathoracic metastatic sites. He received palliative radiation therapy to a total dose of 15 Gy in 5 daily fractions using CT planning and a parallel-opposed pair technique (Figs. 16.3 and 16.4).

A CT scan done approximately 2 months after treatment showed tumor regres-sion and restoration of tracheal and right bronchus patency (Figs. 16.5 and 16.6).

Table 16.1 Mediastinal masses: expected side effects with recommended doses/fractionations

Organ	Side effect	Time of onset	Frequency	Treatment
Kidney	Tumor lysis syndrome	Acute	Associated with large lymphoma tumors	See Chap. 3
Skin	Dryness and skin erythema	Acute effect	Low	Moisturizing cream only is usually sufficient
				Resolves in 2–3 weeks postirradiation
Heart [22–25]	Increased risk of cardiovascular disease	Long-term effect	Low	Adequate long-term follow-up
				Screening and treatment according to guidelines
Thyroid gland [26, 27]	Thyroid dysfunction, mainly hypothyroidism	Long-term effect	Moderate	Adequate long-term follow-up
				Screening and treatment according to guidelines
Other [23, 25, 28]	Increased risk of secondary malignancy	Long-term effect	Low	Adequate long-term follow-up
				Surveillance according to guidelines

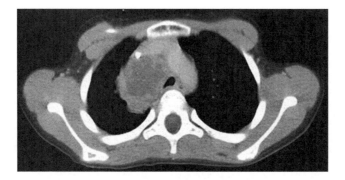

Fig. 16.1 Mediastinal mass compressing trachea before treatment

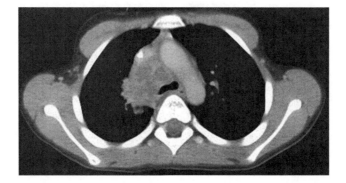

Fig. 16.2 Mediastinal mass compressing trachea before treatment

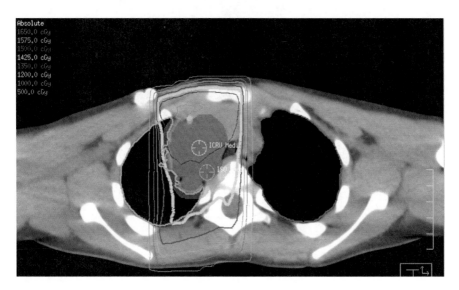

Fig. 16.3 Radiation therapy using parallel-opposed pair technique

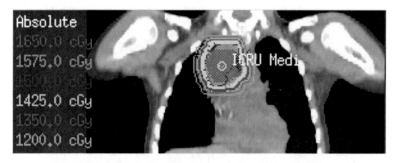

Fig. 16.4 Radiation therapy using parallel-opposed pair technique

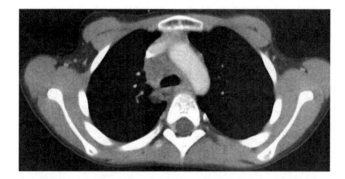

Fig. 16.5 Tumor regression and restoration of tracheal and right bronchus patency

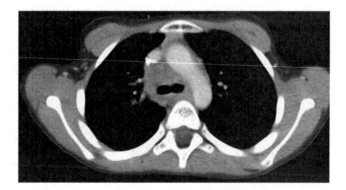

Fig. 16.6 Tumor regression and restoration of tracheal and left bronchus patency

Summary

Urgent mediastinal RT in children is often limited to a small dose (6–7.5 Gy) and relieves symptoms in approximately 75% of patients.

Obtaining a biopsy is always preferable before treating if the diagnosis has not been previously established.

Acute side effects are minor with low doses.

Conformal 3D radiation therapy technique or IMRT should always be the preferred modality if possible.

Abdominal Masses

Symptomatic abdominal masses requiring emergency radiation therapy are mostly seen in the context of infants younger than 1 year old with stage IV-S neuroblastoma and extensive metastatic disease of the liver (i.e., Pepper's syndrome). Marked hepatomegaly can be associated with acute respiratory compromise due to upward pressure on the diaphragm, inferior vena cava obstruction, compromise of renal perfusion, and occasionally gastrointestinal compromise or disseminated intravascular coagulation. In the presence of severe symptomatic hepatomegaly, urgent local abdominal irradiation is indicated, particularly if response to initial chemotherapy has been slow. Less frequently, emergency radiation therapy can also be used to reduce abdominal tumor masses of other histology causing similar severe symptomatology [8]. Details of the differential diagnosis, investigation, and therapy options associated to abdominal masses in children are presented in Chap. 5.

Rationale and Evidence

A few small series describe the role of emergency radiotherapy to palliate abdominal masses. Peschel et al. reported on the high efficacy of radiation therapy for treatment of symptomatic hepatomegaly in three patients with stage IV-S neuroblastoma treated in 1968–1979, and all patients were alive at 2 years after treatment [10]. Blatt et al. reported in 1987 a significant clinical response in seven patients with neuroblastoma and massive hepatomegaly, treated with radiation therapy in 1951–1985 [11]. A modern series by Bertsch et al. [8] reported on the results of urgent abdominal radiation therapy in a heterogeneous group of eight patients treated in 1988–1994 at the Children's Hospital of Philadelphia. The most frequent histology was neuroblastoma, and the main indication for treatment was gastrointestinal obstruction. The response rate to irradiation in this group was 66%.

In evaluating the clinical response to treatment, it is important to keep in mind that symptomatic improvement without measurable change in liver size can occur as early as 2 days after completion of radiation therapy, but complete resolution of hepatomegaly may take up to several months to occur [11].

Technique

The planning procedure is often limited due to the age of the patient and severe symptomatology, particularly in cases with respiratory compromise. For the radiation planning/treatment of young infants, the assistance of an experienced pediatric anesthetic team is necessary. Depending on the severity of respiratory distress, general anesthesia or only sedation may be indicated. CT-based 3D conformal planning is always preferred for readily available treatment. However, since such cases do not generally require high-precision target delineation, clinical markup based on diagnostic imaging and physical exam is also acceptable in some circumstances to expedite treatment. Treatment is given with a parallel-opposed technique using 6-MV photon beams and appropriate shielding. Depending on the clinical response, a total dose of 2–6 Gy, 1.0–1.5 per fraction, is often sufficient to decrease the abdominal burden of disease [9, 11].

Expected Side Effects

Published data on side effects are again based on small series including patients treated with various irradiation techniques and highly variable doses and fractionation schemes [10–12]. In general, acute radiation reactions are minimal with the recommended technique and dose, but prophylactic antiemetic medication administration before treatment avoids the radiation-induced nausea often associated with abdominal irradiation. In terms of late effects, in the series by Blatt et al., at a median follow-up of 8 years, two of the seven irradiated patients had significant late effects. One patient had chondromas in multiple ribs and clinically apparent hypoplasia of the muscles and bones, and the other suffered from radiation nephritis and hepatic fibrosis. However, it was noted by the authors that both patients had been treated before 1970 with radiation doses (>12 Gy) and radiation portals larger than those used in the modern era. Similar findings were described in another series focusing on late toxicity of radiation therapy in 13 neuroblastoma patients with a median follow-up of 23 years. Musculoskeletal toxicity, the most frequent among these patients, was associated with treatment doses exceeding 15 Gy [12]. With the use of lower doses most recently reported, one does not expect to see any liver or renal toxicity and only very minimal late growth effects. There may be a low risk of secondary malignancy in the long term.

Case 2
A 4-month-old infant presented with rapidly increasing abdominal girth and increased respiratory rate. CT imaging showed a right suprarenal mass, a left abdominal mass, and massive hepatomegaly (Figs. 16.7 and 16.8).

Fig. 16.7 CT imaging
showing a right suprarenal
mass, a left abdominal mass,
and massive hepatomegaly
in a 4-month-old infant with
diagnosis of neuroblastoma
stage IV-S

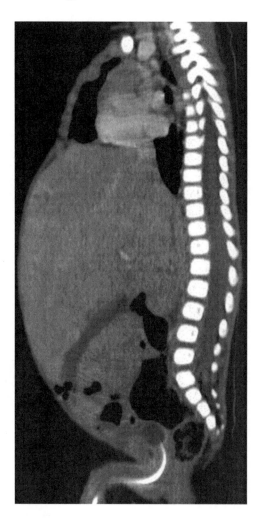

A diagnosis of neuroblastoma stage IV-S was made, and chemotherapy was started. Unfortunately, the patient's respiratory status worsened, and he was referred for emergency radiation therapy of his hepatic disease. A clinical markup with a simple parallel-opposed pair technique (AP/PA fields) (Fig. 16.9) was used.

A total dose of 5 Gy in five daily fractions was delivered. The child had significant clinical improvement 3 weeks after treatment. A progressive resolution of his hepatomegaly was observed as demonstrated on CT scan images at 2 months (Figs. 16.10 and 16.11) and 2.5 years (Figs. 16.12 and 16.13) posttreatment. This patient also received chemotherapy after irradiation and also likely contributed to the hepatic disease response.

Fig. 16.8 CT imaging showing a right suprarenal mass, a left abdominal mass, and massive hepatomegaly in a 4-month-old infant with diagnosis of neuroblastoma stage IV-S

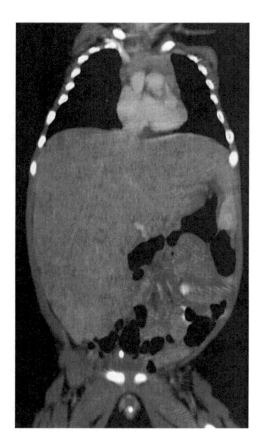

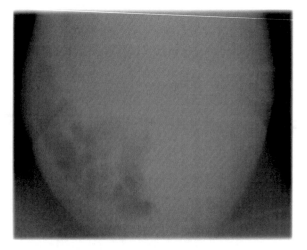

Fig. 16.9 Posterior treatment field

Fig. 16.10 Partial resolution
of hepatomegaly observed 2
months after treatment

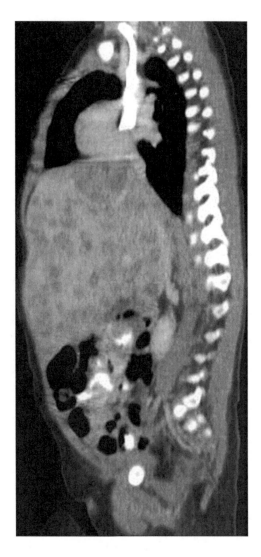

Summary

Stage IV-S neuroblastoma with hepatomegaly is the most common indication for
urgent irradiation in the clinical scenario of an abdominal mass.

Excellent results have been reported in the literature using low total doses of
2–6 Gy.

Clinical markup is still often used in this particular context.

Expected acute and late side effects of this treatment are minimal with the recommended
doses.

Fig. 16.11 Partial resolution
of hepatomegaly observed 2
months after treatment

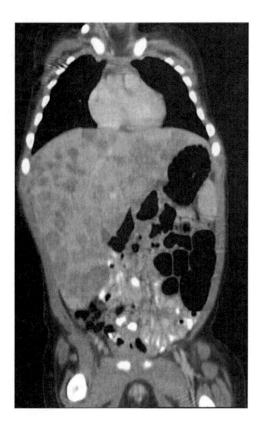

Spinal Cord Compression

Spinal cord compression secondary to primary or metastatic disease is a common indication for emergency radiation therapy in pediatric oncology. Patients must be carefully evaluated clinically and with MRI imaging. High-dose dexamethasone has been demonstrated to be beneficial [13, 14] and should be given to all patients presenting with symptomatic cord compression. Surgical decompression should be considered in patients presenting with spinal instability, bony compression, or paraplegia [14, 15]. This being said, the indication for surgery and/or chemotherapy and/or radiation therapy should be decided on an individual basis by an expert multidisciplinary team. Details of workup, differential diagnosis, and management of this emergency are presented in Chap. 6.

Rationale and Evidence

In the adult population, radiation therapy is well established as an effective modality of emergency treatment for spinal cord compression in combination with

Fig. 16.12 Resolution
of hepatomegaly observed
2.5 years after treatment

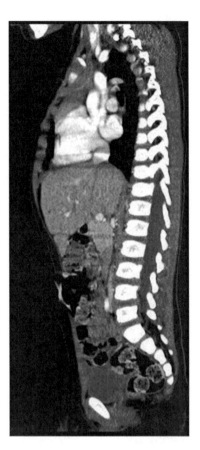

steroids and surgery when indicated [14, 16, 17]. However, in the pediatric population, data on the efficacy of emergency radiation therapy for spinal cord compression are sparse and difficult to interpret. The series reported in the literature are
heterogeneous with various histologies, clinical presentations, and treatment
sequences (steroids/surgery/chemotherapy/radiotherapy). Bertsch et al. reviewed
33 pediatric patients with spinal cord/cauda equina compression or intrinsic cord
lesions treated with urgent RT[8]. The most frequent histology was primitive neu-
roectodermal tumor (PNET), and weakness was the most frequent presenting com-
plaint. The majority of patients (85%) responded to radiotherapy, 55% experiencing
an improvement of their neurologic signs and 30% stabilization. De Bernardi et al.
published on 76 neuroblastoma patients with symptomatic spinal cord compression
at diagnosis [18]. All patients were started on corticosteroid therapy and 11 patients
were treated with radiotherapy. In terms of neurologic outcome in patients who
received RT, 36% recovered, 27% improved, 27% stabilized, while 9% became
worse neurologically.

Fig. 16.13 Resolution
of hepatomegaly observed
2.5 years after treatment

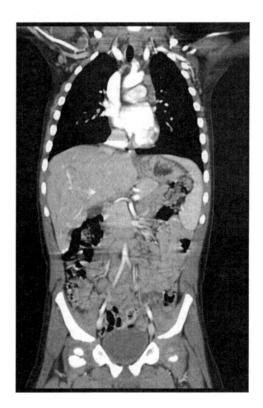

Technique

Whenever possible, diagnostic magnetic resonance imaging should be obtained
to help determine precisely the extension of the lesion causing the spinal cord compression. 3D conformal planning should be used, CT scan imaging notably allowing
a better appreciation of the depth of the lesion and the dose delivered to the spinal
cord. A simple parallel-opposed technique using 6-MV photon beams is most
commonly utilized in this setting. Various dose regimens are used depending
particularly on the histology and location of the tumor, clinical presentation, and in
the context of previous irradiation. Twenty Gy in 5 daily fractions and 30 Gy in 10
daily fractions are commonly used dose regimens.

Expected Side Effects

Very little data are available in the literature to describe the potential side effects of
emergency radiation therapy for spinal cord compression in the pediatric population. Nausea and vomiting can be avoided with the use of appropriate antiemetics

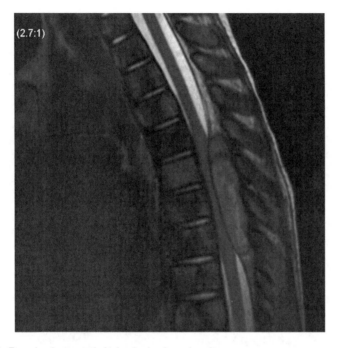

Fig. 16.14 Extradural metastatic lesion in the thoracic spine

prior to each fraction of radiation. Localized erythema and dryness of the skin in the radiation fields can be seen and easily treated with moisturizing cream. Temporary flare-up of pain associated with the lesion can occasionally occur and may be controlled by increased analgesia or corticosteroids.

In terms of subacute/late effects, radiation-induced myelopathy is rarely seen and can usually be avoided by observing known radiation tolerance of the spinal cord. However, exceptional cases of radiation-induced myelopathy can occur even with doses established as within the normal tolerance of the organ. Radiation-induced myelopathy is a diagnosis of exclusion based on many factors including the irradiation dose received by the spinal cord, correlation of symptoms with the region of the cord irradiated, and specific findings on MRI imaging [17]. An expert radiation oncologist should always be involved in the diagnosis and management of any case.

Scoliosis may be a late effect, particularly if prior decompressive surgery has been performed [18, 19].

Case 3

This 6-year-old boy with metastatic neuroblastoma was previously active and suddenly, over 2 days, became unable to move his lower limbs and developed urinary retention. An MRI of spine demonstrated spinal cord compression due to a metastatic intradural extramedullary metastatic lesion in the thoracic spine (Fig. 16.14).

The child was urgently referred to a radiation oncologist, and palliative radiation of 20 Gy/5 fractions to the T5–T9 thoracic levels was planned using CT imaging and a simple parallel-opposed pair technique, with AP/PA fields (Figs. 16.15 and 16.16).

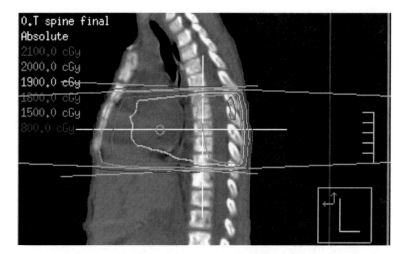

Fig. 16.15 Radiation therapy using a simple parallel-opposed pair technique (AP/PA)

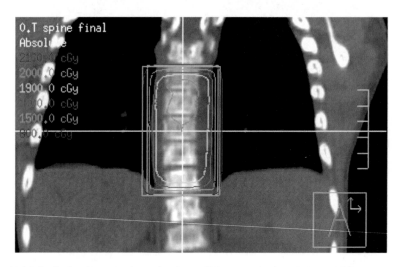

Fig. 16.16 Radiation therapy using a simple parallel-opposed pair technique (AP/PA)

Summary

Every spinal cord compression case should benefit from a multidisciplinary approach in order to determine the best sequence of treatments (steroids and/or surgery and/or chemotherapy and/or radiation therapy).

In general, radiation therapy leads to improvement or stabilization of neurologic symptoms in the majority of patients.

MR imaging of the lesion should be obtained, and conformal 3D radiation therapy techniques should always be preferred.

Significant side effects of irradiation in this context are very rare with standard-dose regimens.

Critical Neurologic Losses

Radiation therapy is a modality which provides a highly effective and rapid locoregional response. When a child is experiencing significant neurologic loss due to tumor progression, radiation therapy is often effective at limiting further loss and can be associated with full recovery in some instances. A classic example is a rapidly progressing skull-base mass compressing the optic structures. Specific histology and clinical presentation varies considerably from one case to another. The opinion of an expert pediatric radiation oncologist should be urgently requested in situations where a child is at significant risk of neurologic loss due to a tumor mass.

Rationale and Evidence

No series of patients have been published regarding this indication. One case report by Kaikov in 1996 described the use of radiation therapy in two pediatric patients with acute leukemia who developed leukemic infiltration of the optic nerve [20]. One patient had her vision saved with the rapid administration of 18 Gy in 10 daily fractions over 2 weeks to the meninges, posterior orbit, and optic nerves.

Technique

The technique and dose are determined individually for each case, and CT simulation and MR imaging are highly valuable. 3D conformal planning is usually mandatory given the proximity of the lesion to the critical neurologic structure. To expedite treatment delivery, a simple technique may be used to deliver the first few fractions of radiation while a more sophisticated plan using IMRT techniques can be developed. IMRT is a more complex and resource-consuming irradiation technique, but allows for better sparing of the surrounding normal tissues (eye structures, optic nerves, optic structures, brain) while achieving highly conformal coverage of the tumor mass.

Expected Side Effects

The possible indication, benefits, and side effects of radiation must be determined individually for each clinical situation. As an illustration, in the case example presented here, expected side effects secondary to irradiation (not secondary to tumor or chemotherapy) are described in Table 16.2 [21].

Case 4

A 7-year-old boy who presented with a short history of plugged nose sensation and rapidly decreasing vision in the left eye. MRI images (Figs. 16.17 and 16.18) documented a large nasopharynx/nasal mass that was invading the skull base and extending into the left orbital apex region, accounting for his significant loss of visual fields on the left side.

A transnasal biopsy confirmed a nasopharyngeal embryonal rhabdomyosarcoma. Radiation therapy was started urgently the following morning. Treatment was first planned using 3D conformal planning, and a fusion of CT scan images with MR images was done. A parallel-opposed photon beam technique (Figs. 16.19–16.21) was used for the first five fractions. This technique gave sufficient tumor coverage while allowing for rapid delivery of radiotherapy in the context of visual loss secondary to the growing nasopharyngeal tumor. Then, during the first days of treatment, a second plan using IMRT was developed (Figs. 16.22 and 16.23) and replaced the 3D conformal plan after five treatments. The patient received more than 80% of his irradiation via IMRT, limiting the normal tissue exposure of this treatment. A total dose of 50.4 Gy in 28 daily fractions was delivered.

A follow-up CT scan 1 year after treatment (Fig. 16.24) showed complete resolution of the mass. The patient has had some improvement in his visual symptoms, but vision remains impaired.

Summary

Radiation therapy can provide a highly effective and rapid local and locoregional response, and this can be very useful in certain clinical settings to avoid critical neurologic loss.

A classic example is a rapidly progressing mass compressing the optic apparatus.

The opinion of an expert pediatric radiation oncologist should be requested in situations where a child could suffer a significant neurologic loss due to a tumor mass.

The possible indication, benefit, and side effects of an irradiation in this context will be determined individually for each clinical situation.

Table 16.2 Critical neurologic losses: expected side effects in the presented case example

Organ	Side effect	Time of onset	Frequency	Treatment
Skin	Dryness and skin erythema	Acute side effect	Moderate	Moisturizing cream only is usually sufficient
				Resolves in 2–3 weeks postirradiation
Hair	Patchy loss of hair corresponding to the entry and exit portals of the radiation beams	Acute side effect	High	None, hair will regrow spontaneously in 2–3 months following the end of radiation therapy in most areas
Nasal/sinus mucosa	Dryness, erythema, and excessive secretions	Acute and subacute side effect	High	Regular irrigation of nose with saline solution
	Possible epistaxis			Pain medication if needed
				Excessive secretions can persist for a few months after treatment
Oral mucosa (palate)	Possible temporary xerostomia, erythema of mucosa, and possible ulceration	Acute side effect	Moderate	Analgesic mouthwash per oral pain medication if needed
				Soft diet and dietician follow-up if needed
				Regular follow-up of the patient's weight
				Symptoms will resolve in the weeks following end of treatment
Eyes (conjunctiva)	Erythema and dryness of the conjunctiva	Acute	Low to moderate	Artificial tears/ointment for comfort
				Symptoms will resolve in the weeks following the end of treatment
General status	Increased fatigue	Acute and subacute side effect	High	No treatment
				Will resolve in the weeks to months following irradiation
Bones/muscles	Moderate effect on future growth based on the age of the patient and dose/fractionation	Long-term effect		Adequate follow-up
	Possible facial hypoplasia/asymmetry			Surgical intervention if needed

(continued)

Table 16.2 (continued)

Organ	Side effect	Time of onset	Frequency	Treatment
Teeth	Impact on future teeth growth	Long-term effect	Moderate	Adequate follow-up in collaboration with a pediatric dentist specialized in oncology Intervention if needed
Parotid	Xerostomia	Acute, subacute and/ or long-term effect	Low to moderate	Referral to a pediatric dentist specialized in oncology
Pituitary hormones deficiency	Growth hormone and thyroid hormone are the most likely to be affected	Long-term effect	Moderate	Adequate regular follow-up in collaboration with a pediatric endocrinologist
	FSH and LH hormones could also be affected			Hormone replacement if needed
Eye (lenses)	Development of bilateral cataracts	Long-term effect	High	Adequate follow-up Cataract extraction if symptomatic
Other [23, 25]	Increased risk of secondary malignancies	Long-term effect	Low	Follow-up in a long-term effects clinic Surveillance according to guidelines

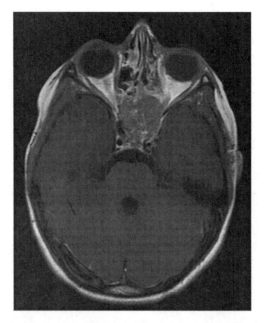

Fig. 16.17 Large nasopharynx/nasal embryonal rhabdomyosarcoma invading the skull base and extending into the left orbital apex region

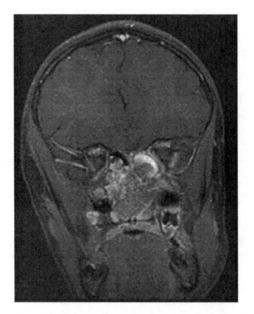

Fig. 16.18 Large nasopharynx/nasal embryonal rhabdomyosarcoma invading the skull base and extending into the left orbital apex region

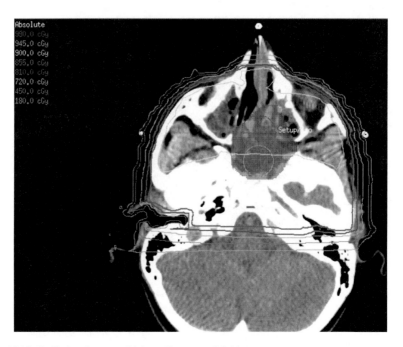

Fig. 16.19 Radiation therapy with laterally opposed fields

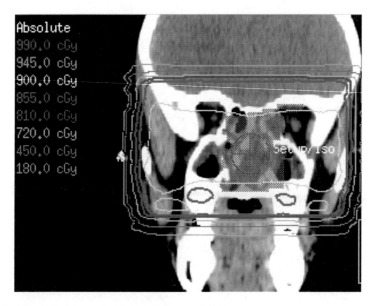

Fig. 16.20 Radiation therapy with laterally opposed fields

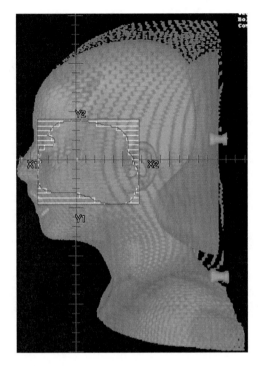

Fig. 16.21 Radiation therapy with laterally opposed fields

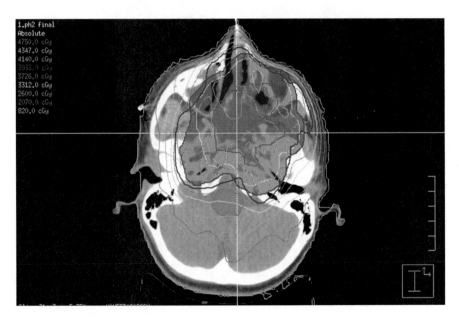

Fig. 16.22 Radiation therapy using IMRT planning technique

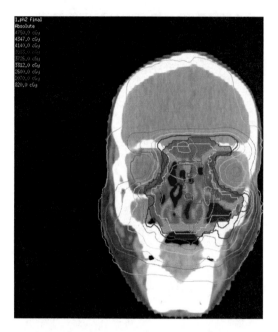

Fig. 16.23 Radiation therapy using IMRT planning technique

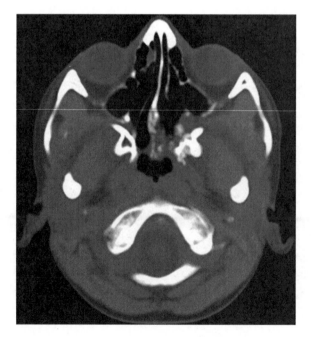

Fig. 16.24 Follow-up CT scan 1 year after treatment showing complete resolution of the mass

The technique can vary depending on the precise context, but 3D conformal planning is usually mandatory given the proximity of the lesion to the critical neurologic structure.

Conclusion

Radiotherapy can be a beneficial and efficacious treatment in the context of pediatric oncological emergencies, with the potential of providing rapid tumor response and decompression of critical structures.

References

1. Hall, E.J., Radiobiology for the radiologist. 6th ed. Philadelphia: Lippincott Williams & Wilkins. 2006; 546.
2. Khan, F.M., The Physics of Radiation Therapy. 3rd ed. Philadelphia: Lippincott Williams & Wilkins. 2003; 560.
3. Loeffler, J.S., et al., Emergency prebiopsy radiation for mediastinal masses: impact on subsequent pathologic diagnosis and outcome. J Clin Oncol, 1986. 4(5): p. 716–21.
4. Davenport, D., et al., Response of superior vena cava syndrome to radiation therapy. Cancer, 1976; 38(4): p. 1577–80.
5. Armstrong, B.A., et al., Role of irradiation in the management of superior vena cava syndrome. Int J Radiat Oncol Biol Phys, 1987; 13(4): p. 531–9.
6. Egelmeers, A., et al., Palliative effectiveness of radiation therapy in the treatment of superior vena cava syndrome. Bull Cancer Radiother, 1996; 83(3): p. 153–7.
7. Rowell, N.P. and F.V. Gleeson, Steroids, radiotherapy, chemotherapy and stents for superior vena caval obstruction in carcinoma of the bronchus: a systematic review. Clin Oncol (R Coll Radiol), 2002; 14(5): p. 338–51.
8. Bertsch, H., et al., Emergent/urgent therapeutic irradiation in pediatric oncology: patterns of presentation, treatment, and outcome. Med Pediatr Oncol, 1998; 30(2): p. 101–5.
9. Halperin, E.C., Pediatric Radiation Oncology. 4th ed. Philadelphia, PA: Lippincott Williams & Wilkins. 2005; 676.
10. Peschel, R.E., M. Chen, and J. Seashore, The treatment of massive hepatomegaly in stage IV-S neuroblastoma. Int J Radiat Oncol Biol Phys, 1981; 7(4): p. 549–53.
11. Blatt, J., M. Deutsch, and M.R. Wollman, Results of therapy in stage IV-S neuroblastoma with massive hepatomegaly. Int J Radiat Oncol Biol Phys, 1987; 13(10): p. 1467–71.
12. Paulino, A.C., et al., Locoregional control in infants with neuroblastoma: role of radiation therapy and late toxicity. Int J Radiat Oncol Biol Phys, 2002; 52(4): p. 1025–31.
13. Sorensen, S., et al., Effect of high-dose dexamethasone in carcinomatous metastatic spinal cord compression treated with radiotherapy: a randomised trial. Eur J Cancer, 1994; 30A(1): p. 22–7.
14. Loblaw, D.A. and N.J. Laperriere, Emergency treatment of malignant extradural spinal cord compression: an evidence-based guideline. J Clin Oncol, 1998; 16(4): p. 1613–24.
15. Patchell, R.A., et al., Direct decompressive surgical resection in the treatment of spinal cord compression caused by metastatic cancer: a randomised trial. Lancet, 2005; 366(9486): p. 643–8.

16. Loblaw, D.A., et al., Systematic review of the diagnosis and management of malignant extradural spinal cord compression: the Cancer Care Ontario Practice Guidelines Initiative's Neuro-Oncology Disease Site Group. J Clin Oncol, 2005; 23(9): p. 2028–37.

17. Gunderson, L.L. and J.E. Tepper, Clinical Radiation Oncology. 2nd ed. Philadelphia, PA: Elsevier Churchill Livingstone. 2007; 1827.

18. De Bernardi, B., et al., Neuroblastoma with symptomatic spinal cord compression at diagnosis: treatment and results with 76 cases. J Clin Oncol, 2001; 19(1): p. 183–90.

19. Poretti, A., et al., Long-term complications and quality of life in children with intraspinal tumors. Pediatr Blood Cancer, 2008; 50(4): p. 844–8.

20. Kaikov, Y., Optic nerve head infiltration in acute leukemia in children: an indication for emergency optic nerve radiation therapy. Med Pediatr Oncol, 1996; 26(2): p. 101–4.

21. Raney, R.B., et al., Late complications of therapy in 213 children with localized, nonorbital soft-tissue sarcoma of the head and neck: A descriptive report from the Intergroup Rhabdomyosarcoma Studies (IRS)-II and - III. IRS Group of the Children's Cancer Group and the Pediatric Oncology Group. Med Pediatr Oncol, 1999; 33(4): p. 362–71.

22. Adams, M.J., et al., Radiation-associated cardiovascular disease. Crit Rev Oncol Hematol, 2003; 45(1): p. 55–75.

23. Landier, W., W.H. Wallace, and M.M. Hudson, Long-term follow-up of pediatric cancer survivors: education, surveillance, and screening. Pediatr Blood Cancer, 2006; 46(2): p. 149–58.

24. Shankar, S.M., et al., Monitoring for cardiovascular disease in survivors of childhood cancer: report from the Cardiovascular Disease Task Force of the Children's Oncology Group. Pediatrics, 2008; 121(2): p. e387–96.

25. Landier, W., et al., Development of risk-based guidelines for pediatric cancer survivors: the Children's Oncology Group Long-Term Follow-Up Guidelines from the Children's Oncology Group Late Effects Committee and Nursing Discipline. J Clin Oncol, 2004; 22(24): p. 4979–90.

26. Peerboom, P.F., et al., Thyroid function 10–18 years after mantle field irradiation for Hodgkin's disease. Eur J Cancer, 1992; 28A(10): p. 1716–8.

27. Constine, L.S., et al., Thyroid dysfunction after radiotherapy in children with Hodgkin's disease. Cancer, 1984; 53(4): p. 878–83.

28. Robison, L.L., et al., Long-term outcomes of adult survivors of childhood cancer. Cancer, 2005; 104(11 Suppl): p. 2557–64.

Index

Printed by Publishers' Graphics LLC
DBT130808.15.16.2